Student Learning Guide to accompany

MOSBY'S

Pharmacology in Nursing

21st Edition

Leda M. McKenry, PhD, CRN, FNP, FAAN
Evelyn Salerno, RPh, BS, PharmD, FASCP

Student Learning Guide prepared by

Jane M. Hartsock, RN, MA, AOCN
Formerly, Associate Professor
Trinity College of Nursing
Moline, Illinois

Acknowledgments for Past Contributors

Linda K. Wendling, MA
Golden M. Tradewell, MSN, MA, RN

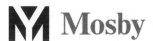 Mosby

An Imprint of Elsevier Science
St. Louis   London   Philadelphia   Sydney   Toronto

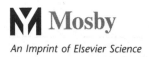

An Imprint of Elsevier Science

Vice President & Publishing Director, Nursing: Sally Schrefer
Executive Editor: Robin Carter
Managing Editor: Lee Henderson
Cover Design: Bill Drone
Project Manager: Gayle Morris
Manufacturing Supervisor: Maureen Niebruegge

NOTICE

Pharmacology is an ever-changing field. Standard safety precautions must be followed, but as new research and clinical experience broaden our knowledge, changes in treatment and drug therapy may become necessary or appropriate. Readers are advised to check the most current product information provided by the manufacturer of each drug to be administered to verify the recommended dose, the method and duration of administration, and contraindications. It is the responsibility of the licensed prescriber relying on experience and knowledge of the patient, to determine dosages and the best treatment for each individual patient. Neither the publisher nor the editor assumes any liability for any injury and/or damage to persons or property arising from this publication.

ISBN: 0-323-01006-7

02 03 04 FG/EB 9 8 7 6 5 4 3 2

Chapter 1   Orientation to Pharmacology

1. Match the person or groups to the historical event that best relates to them.

   ____ Asclepios

   ____ Religious orders

   ____ Arabs

   ____ Valerius Cordus

   ____ Codex

   ____ Hippocrates

   ____ Paracelsus

   a. First important national pharmacopeia, from France

   b. Formulated first set of drug standards

   c. Wrote first pharmacopeia

   d. Greek god of healing

   e. Believed diseases resulted from natural causes

   f. Aided sick and needy with good food and rest

   g. Denounced "humoral pathology" and substituted actual diseases with specific remedies

2. Using your text, the *Physician's Desk Reference,* and the *Hospital Formulary,* look up the following drugs and give their official, generic, trade, and chemical names.

	Official name	**Generic name**	**Trade name**	**Chemical name**
Aspirin				
Chlorothiazide				
Diazepam				
Ethacrynic acid				

3. List the five steps of the nursing process.

4. Cryptoquote: The cryptoquote is a substitution cipher in which one letter stands for another. If you think that Y equals an A, than every Y in the sentence is an A. Look for one- and two-letter words to begin to decipher the sentence, then look for patterns of letters until you solve the puzzle.

   Clue: A = M

   Fekcm hsf uhyom cr islgaldcncbm!

Chapter 2   Legal and Ethical Aspects of Medication Administration

1. Match the law/act to the definition that best describes it.

   ____ Pure Food and Drug Act (1906)

   ____ Sherley Amendment (1912)

   ____ Food, Drug and Cosmetic Act (1938)

   ____ Durkham-Humphrey Amendment (1952)

   ____ Controlled Substances Act (1970)

   a. Increased research into, prevention of, and treatment for drug abuse

   b. First federal law to protect the public from mislabeled drugs

   c. Related to prescription of drugs and refills

   d. Prevented marketing new drugs before they were properly tested

   e. Prohibited the use of fraudulent therapeutic claims

2. Indicate whether the following are true (**T**) or false (**F**).

   ____ A category X drug indicates that the drug causes fetal abnormalities.

   ____ A category B drug indicates that it is safe to give the drug to a pregnant woman.

   ____ A schedule V drug indicates that a drug may be sold without a prescription.

   ____ A category D drug indicates that a drug may have possible risk to a human fetus.

3. List three conditions that should be present before a nurse can legally administer a medication.

4. Word search:

FDA	NARCOTICS	SAFEGUARDS
INVESTIGATIONAL	NURSING	STANDARDS
LEGEND	ORDERS	TOXICITY
LEGISLATION	PRESCRIPTION	

```
J  L  F  L  M  I  N  V  E  S  T  I  G  A  T  I  O  N  A  L
N  E  K  D  D  J  Q  B  A  J  K  S  R  E  D  R  O  A  L  R
M  G  K  Y  A  F  P  F  T  N  R  M  I  R  M  I  E  R  C  W
Z  E  A  W  S  X  E  O  Y  U  K  K  I  I  T  S  U  C  K  I
B  N  T  P  Q  G  X  M  O  R  T  R  P  A  T  B  N  O  I  D
D  D  Q  P  U  I  A  Z  U  S  J  Q  L  A  G  B  F  T  Z  A
V  Q  M  A  C  W  C  H  T  I  C  S  N  S  Y  N  E  I  J  P
Y  Z  R  I  J  L  M  I  Q  N  I  D  T  U  X  K  C  C  K  E
E  D  T  V  U  B  G  I  D  G  A  M  G  F  M  B  I  S  M  U
S  Y  H  B  V  Q  X  T  E  R  B  P  G  T  R  X  M  Z  W  C
B  I  Z  I  O  A  K  L  D  X  H  S  Q  M  F  P  O  J  N  Y
F  L  T  I  P  R  E  S  C  R  I  P  T  I  O  N  Z  G  M  I
```

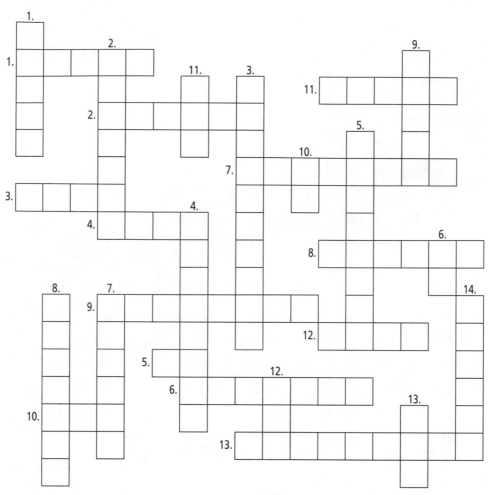

Across

1. A way to administer medications
2. Liquid part of the blood
3. A factor affecting the dose of medications for a child
4. Area in which inhalants are absorbed
5. The abbreviation for therapeutic index
6. A form in which a drug can be taken orally
7. Objective and subjective effects of a drug
8. Environment that increases the absorption of aspirin
9. Movement of a drug in the body is called pharmaco-_____.
10. Factor affecting the effects of a drug
11. Organic substance insoluble in water
12. Fundamental unit of all living organisms
13. Term for process of ridding the body of a drug

Down

1. Another term for medications
2. Route in which medications are applied to the skin
3. Adverse reaction produced unintentionally
4. Factors we are born with that can affect drug effects
5. Smallest amount of a substance that can exist alone
6. Abbreviation for route in which a drug is instilled into muscle
7. Organ that can eliminate drugs
8. Organ that aids in absorption of a drug
9. Various places where drugs can be injected
10. Abbreviation for route in which a drug is instilled into tissue
11. Abbreviation for aspirin
12. Factor affecting the metabolism of a drug
13. Form in which a drug can be applied to the skin
14. Pharmacodynamics of a drug

Chapter 4   Assessment, Nursing Diagnosis, and Planning

1. For each of the items listed below, indicate what part of the nursing process describes this nursing activity. Write an **A** for assessment, **D** for diagnosis, **P** for planning, **I** for implementation, and **E** for evaluation.

_____ Chief complaint of the patient

_____ Checking arm band or ID tag before drug administration

_____ Nausea related to chemotherapy

_____ Recording secondary effects

_____ Noncompliance with prescribed steroid therapy

_____ Monitoring therapeutic response to a drug

_____ History of allergy

_____ Behavioral objectives for the client

_____ Instillation of eye drops

_____ Calculating flow rate for oxygen therapy

_____ Vital signs

_____ Observing a client demonstrate proper self-medication with insulin

_____ Conversion of an apothecary measure to metric while transcribing a medication order

2. Explain the following drug orders. Classify the order as a routine order **(RO)**, stat order **(Stat)**, prn order **(prn)**, or single order **(S)**.

Classification	Explanation of Drug Order

a._____   Demerol 100 mg IM stat_____

b._____   MOM 30 ml po h.s. _____

c._____   Seconal 100 mg po h.s. p.r.n._____

d. _____   Lanoxin 0.25 mg po qd_____

e. _____   Dilantin 100 mg po_____

3. Mr. Jones develops an elevated temperature. The doctor orders "ASA gr x po stat." Identify the following client reactions as either a therapeutic response to the medication **(T)**, an allergic reaction **(A)**, or a side effect/adverse reaction **(S)**.

_____ Mr. Jones develops shortness of breath.

_____ Temperature returns to normal.

_____ Mr. Jones complains of stomach ache.

4. For collaborative problems, the nurse's responsibility is to _____, _____, and _____.

Chapter 5   Implementation and Evaluation

1. The following abbreviations are commonly used in relation to medication administration. Match the definition to the term it best describes.

_____ ac	a. Before meals
	b. After meals
_____ bid	c. Drops
	d. Ointment
_____ gtts	e. Right eye
	f. By mouth
_____ os	g. Two times per day
	h. Three times per day
_____ qid	i. 8:00 AM, noon, 4:00 PM, 8:00 PM
	j. 9:00 AM daily
_____ tid	k. 9:00 AM, 1:00 PM, 6:00 PM
	l. Each eye
_____ qd	
_____ ou	

2. 1 tbsp = _____ oz = _____ dram = _____ ml

3. 1 glassful = _____ ml = _____ oz

4. 3 tsp = _____ gtts

5. 0.5 gm = _____ mg

6. 2000 ml = _____ L

7. _____ drams = gr ix

8. 100 mg = _____ gm

9. 1 mg = _____ micrograms

10. _____ oz = 1 lb

11. 120 grains = _____ drams

12. 164 kg = _____ lb

13. 64 gal = _____ L

14. 6 cm = _____ m

15. Calculate the following problems for parenteral dosages.

    a. Morphine sulfate 10 mg
        Available: Morphine sulfate 16 mg/ml

    b. Desired: Penicillin G 400,000 U IM
        Available: Penicillin G 1,000,000 U in 5 ml

    c. Desired: Atropine sulfate gr 1/150
        Available: Atropine sulfate 0.6 mg/ml

16. Infuse 500 ml blood in 2 hours. Administration set has a drop factor of 10. How many drops/min?

17. Client was given 1000 ml NS in 5 hours. What was the rate of administration (flow rate) if the drop factor was 15?

18. No sustained-action drug form should be _____ or vigorously mixed with food for administration.

19. Amber-colored containers protect some medications against _____ by light.

20. Narcotic drugs must be kept in a _____ and _____ at the end of a shift.

Chapter 6   Cultural and Psychologic Aspects of Drug Therapy

1. Match the listed cultural group to the values statement at the left. There may be more than one answer for each values statement.

____ Belief in hot-cold therapy

____ Technology dependent

____ God's will must prevail

____ Rhythmicity

____ Patriarchal

____ Music and physical activities

____ Extended family valued

____ Folk foods

a. African-American

b. Mexican-American

c. Anglo-American

d. Haitian-American

e. North American Indian

2. List three primary methods of traditional Chinese healing.

3. Word search:

AFRICAN	FOLK	NATIVE
AMERICANS	HAITIAN	RELIGION
ASIAN	HARMONY	SPIRITUAL
CULTURE	HISPANIC	

```
Y A C U L T U R E Q N P
M M F O L K N N J O S O
U E D R B A A Q I E P X
M R L Z I T S G Q N I U
S I C T I C I H E C R B
B C I V A L A G I I I K
S A E H E R N N J M T U
H N F R M S A G P D U P
L S N O G P N K X M A O
I I N F S M I Y M X L Z
W Y K I E L D K I L N Y
J Q H Z E B G J B K M Z
```

Chapter 7   Maternal and Child Drug Therapy

1. Describe how ear drops should be administered to a child.

2. Calculate the following dosages for children using the different rules and the nomogram for determining body surface area for children.

Adult dose	Age of child	Weight (lb)	Height (in)	Clark	BSA
Atropine sulfate gr 1/150	18 mo	25	32		
Aminophylline 0.5 gm	6 yr	38	42		
Gentamycin 80 mg	22 mo	28	33		

3. Jumbled words:

   a. This protects the fetus from receiving drugs in the maternal circulation.

      CANPTEAL_____

   b. These enable the nurse to meet the goal of protecting the mother while promoting the role of the family.

      ACLABNE DAN VADTEACO_____

4. Match the nursing interventions at the left to the developmental age.

   _____ Perform the procedure swiftly, then comfort   a. Infants

   _____ Encourage self-expression and self-care   b. Toddlers

   _____ Offer concrete explanation and perform   c. Preschoolers
         quickly
                                                            d. School-aged children
   _____ Explain how the medication works
                                                            e. Adolescents
   _____ Make use of magical thinking

   _____ Allow self-comforting measures

   _____ Use play for expression of feelings

Chapter 8   Drug Therapy for Older Adults

1. List physiologic factors affecting pharmacokinetics in the older adult.

2. List some factors that may complicate drug therapy in the older adult.

3. How can a nurse reduce or eliminate the potentially adverse risk factors associated with various drug regimens?

4. What steps should the nurse take in educating the client regarding medication administration?

5. Unscramble the letters for the words below and enter them in the proper places in the scrabble grid from top to bottom.

NUFCONIT, DARCCAI TPUOTOU, DOLOB WLOF, NRISDOUITIBT, VRELI, MALBIUN, PHACAIT.
PTNOBASOIR, CRETNSAIO, NALE SMAS, XCEIETONR, IG YILOIMTT, DYKIEN, TREAW YBDO, LBOSMITEAM, SPAS
TSFIR, KNEICOPMCSOHRA, PCOSMIINOTO, SOSL, HP CGTAISR, CCHMEOOYRT, AFT ROSTSE, SDEECDRAE.

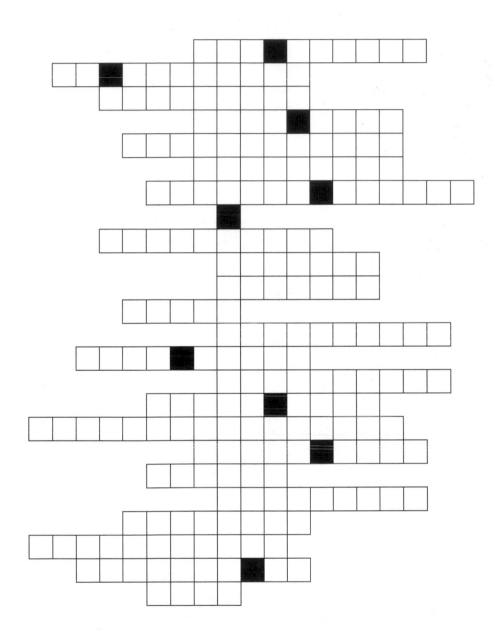

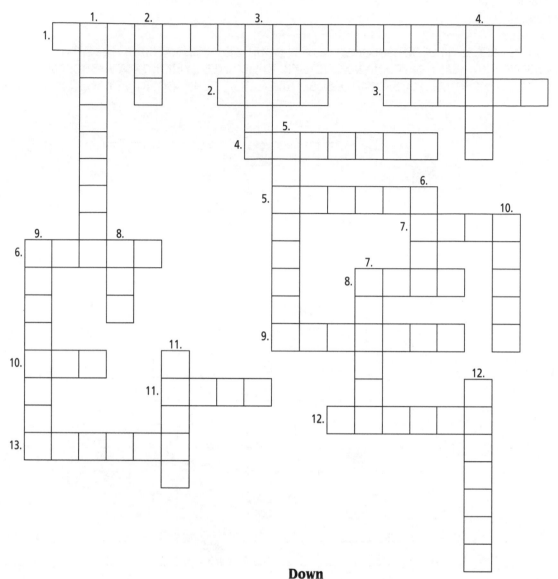

Across

1. Emotional reliance on a drug
2. Initials for federal agency that monitors data on drug abuse
3. Indiscriminate use of drugs
4. Many _____ remedies contain alcohol
5. Sign of drug intoxication with barbiturates
6. Amphetamines are often called pep _____
7. Possible result of acute overdose of opiates
8. Alcoholic beverage often abused by teenagers
9. Related to the belladonna alkaloids
10. Phencyclidine
11. Person can do this if he or she stops abusing
12. Frequently abused OTC drug
13. Pinpoint pupil

Down

1. Combination of heroin and cocaine
2. Few drugs without these effects are abused
3. Severe toxicity can lead to this
4. Form of cannabis
5. Often abused by young athletes
6. Adverse effect of steroid use by females
7. An alcoholic beverage
8. A hallucinogenic drug
9. Continuing erections
10. Drug use leading to dependence
11. Effect of IV injection of amphetamines
12. Effect of cocaine

1. Word search:

ASSESSMENT	IMPLEMENTATION	PLANNING
BARRIERS	LANGUAGE	READINESS
COMPLIANCE	LEARNING	TEACHING
DEVELOPMENTAL	MEMORY	THOUGHT
ERIKSON	MONITORING	VERBS
EVALUATION	NURSING	VISION
HEARING	PERCEPTION	

```
T  G  J  O  U  P  L  A  N  N  I  N  G  A
H  H  N  X  T  X  U  X  Y  K  R  K  N  L
L  N  O  I  T  P  E  C  R  E  P  K  I  K
M  V  N  U  R  S  I  N  G  S  J  R  H  O
R  P  F  O  G  O  D  R  T  O  B  X  C  Z
R  A  T  P  O  H  T  D  D  W  Q  R  A  A
L  N  N  O  K  W  T  I  F  W  Z  E  E  P
A  S  S  E  S  S  M  E  N  T  C  D  T  V
N  B  A  R  R  I  E  R  S  O  G  H  R  J
O  H  C  W  M  P  L  Q  M  L  M  T  E  D
I  D  E  V  E  L  O  P  M  E  N  T  A  L
T  B  F  A  B  B  L  B  R  A  H  P  D  A
A  Y  M  V  R  I  S  I  C  R  S  N  I  N
U  J  J  E  A  I  K  V  N  N  O  Z  N  G
L  G  X  N  M  S  N  U  X  I  P  B  E  U
A  R  C  U  O  O  Q  G  S  N  E  B  S  A
V  E  Q  N  A  L  R  I  U  G  Y  S  S  G
E  D  E  U  N  Q  V  Y  M  O  M  W  U  E
I  M  P  L  E  M  E  N  T  A  T  I  O  N
```

2. List factors that can foster noncompliance or ineffective management of the therapeutic regimen.

3. Write two measurable goals for a client learning to self-administer medications.

4. Match Erickson's stage of development to tasks to be accomplished.

_____ Infant   a. Identity vs role confusion

_____ Toddler   b. Trust vs mistrust

_____ Preschooler   c. Generativity vs stagnation

_____ Adolescent   d. Initiative vs guilt

_____ Middle-aged adult   e. Autonomy vs shame

_____ Older adult   f. Integrity vs despair

Chapter 11   Over-the-Counter Medications

1. Define the following words:

   a. Analgesic_____

   b. Constipation_____

   c. Perceived constipation_____

2. Describe GRASE.

3. List important information to teach clients about OTC use of aspirin.

4. Match the laxative in the left column to its type.

   ____ Psyllium

   ____ Mineral oil

   ____ Docusate

   ____ Magnesium hydroxide

   ____ Senna

   ____ Effervescent sodium phosphate

   ____ Castor oil

   ____ Bisacodyl

   ____ Polycarbophil calcium

   ____ Cascara sagrada

   a. Saline

   b. Stimulant

   c. Bulk forming

   d. Lubricant

   e. Emollient

5. Describe the action of adsorbent antidiarrheals.

6. List side/adverse reactions of decongestants.

Chapter 12   Complementary and Alternative Pharmacology

1. Match the therapeutic effects to the herbal remedies.

   ____ Prevents liver damage

   ____ Active against intestinal parasites

   ____ Increases cells in bone marrow

   ____ Promotes sleep

   ____ Stimulates interferon production

   ____ Decreases serum cholesterol

   ____ Effective for osteoarthritis and rheumatoid arthritis

   ____ Has multiple pharmacologic actions including antitumor activity

   ____ Relieves headache

   ____ Increases cardiac contractility

   a. Astragalus

   b. Echinacea

   c. Feverfew

   d. Garlic

   e. Ginger

   f. Ginseng root

   g. Green tea

   h. Hawthorne

   i. Milk thistle

   j. Stark cartilage

   k. Valerian

2. Develop a teaching plan for a client taking Lobelia to help stop smoking.

3. Cryptoquote: The cryptoquote is a substitute cipher in which one letter stands for another. If you think that Y equals an A, than every Y in the sentence is an A. Look for one- and two-letter words to decipher the sentence, then look for patterns of letters until you solve the puzzle.

   Clue: O = P

   EATIAOSMEU CB S BUBMIT AD MEIFSOIYMCNB

Chapter 13   Overview of the Central Nervous System

1. The blood-brain barrier is a covering of _____ (called _____) that encircle_____.

2. The extrapyramidal system is _____; it is associated with _____.

3. The primary functions of the reticular activating system are _____, _____, and _____.

4. The best known chemical transmitter of nerve impulses is _____.

5. Endorphins suppress _____.

6. An increase in catecholamines and serotonin causes _____.

7. The _____ controls memory storage and motor functions.

8. The _____ registers such sensations as pain and temperature.

9. The hypothalamus is a major link between the _____ and the _____.

10. The midbrain, pons, and medulla oblongata comprise the _____.

11. The two major cell types in the CNS are _____ and _____.

12. List three catecholamines and their effects on the central nervous system.

13. On the drawing below, identify and label the following:

    1. Synaptic vesicles
    2. Cell body
    3. Mitochondria
    4. Golgi
    5. Nerve terminals
    6. Dendrites
    7. Axon
    8. Nucleus
    9. Rough endoplasmic reticulum
    10. Nissl body

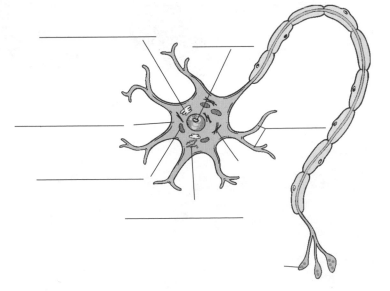

Chapter 14   Analgesics

1. List some of the more serious adverse reactions reported with morphine.

2. What is the recommended treatment for aspirin overdose?

3. Describe briefly the three steps recommended for pain management according to severity of pain.

4. Label the opiods that bind with the receptors shown:

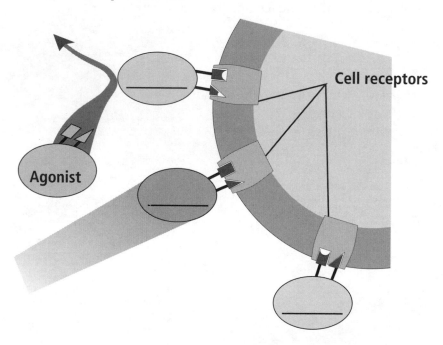

Chapter 15   Anesthetics

1. The two major categories of anesthesia are general and _____ or _____.

2. The advantage of balanced anesthesia is _____.

3. Malignant hyperthermia is a dangerous adverse effect of _____, _____ anesthetics.

4. Dissociative anesthesia produces _____ and _____ but not _____.

5. Match the physiologic effect to the stage of anesthesia in which it occurs.

   _____ Vivid dreams

   _____ Numbness

   _____ Rapid eye movement

   _____ Lowered body temperature

   _____ Exaggerated reflexes

   _____ Laughter

   _____ Shallow respiration

   _____ Vasomotor collapse

   a. Analgesia

   b. Excitement

   c. Surgical anesthesia

   d. Medullary paralysis (toxic stage)

6. Develop a nursing diagnosis, goal, and interventions for an elderly client receiving a general anesthetic.

Chapter 16   Antianxiety, Sedative, and Hypnotic Drugs

1. Antianxiety or anxiolytic agents are used to _____.

2. Sedatives and hypnotics are _____ drugs. The major difference between them is the degree of _____ induced.

3. REM (rapid eye movement) sleep is also referred to as _____ or _____ sleep.

4. Insomnia is a frequent concern of _____.

5. List data necessary to collect from a client receiving sedatives/hypnotics during the assessment phase of the nursing process.

6. Develop a care plan (nursing diagnosis, goal, and interventions) for a pediatric client receiving an antianxiety drug.

7. What are nonpharmacologic approaches the client may take to try to resolve insomnia?

1. What is the physiologic mechanism producing the symptoms of epilepsy?

2. Name two adverse reactions of barbiturates.

3. Hydantoins are commonly used for the treatment of _____.

4. Indicate whether the following are true **(T)** or false **(F)**.

   _____ Barbiturates are classed as anticonvulsants and so are not a controlled substance.

   _____ Elderly clients are less sensitive to barbiturates and can tolerate higher dosages.

   _____ Hydantoins are noted for their lack of drug interactions.

5. Develop a nursing care plan (nursing diagnosis, goals, and interventions) for a child receiving an anticonvulsant.

6. Match the anticonvulsant to the side effects associated with it.

   _____ Apnea, laryngospasm   a. Phenobarbital

   _____ Ataxia, drowsiness   b. Phenytoin

   _____ Hiccups, headaches   c. Diazepam

   _____ Hirsutism, gingival hyperplasia   d. Ethosuximide

Chapter 18   Central Nervous System Stimulants

1. Amphetamines are mainly stimulants of the _____.

2. ADD with hyperactivity is a syndrome characterized by _____, _____, _____, and _____.

3. For clients with narcolepsy, CNS stimulants are useful in controlling _____ and _____.

4. Cataplexy is generalized _____ associated with _____.

5. Hypnagogic illusions are _____.

6. List important concepts to teach the client who is receiving amphetamines.

7. List side effects of methylphenidate hydrochloride.

8. Describe at least one effect of caffeine on each of the various body systems.

   Neurologic_____

   Autonomic nervous system_____

   Cardiac_____

   Vascular_____

   Renal_____

   Gastrointestinal_____

   Sensory_____

   Pulmonary_____

1. Match each drug with its classification.

    ____ chlorpromazine   a. MAO inhibitors

    ____ isocarboxazid   b. Tricyclic antidepressants

    ____ Eskalith   c. Phenothiazine derivatives

    ____ Prozac   d. Lithium

    ____ amitriptyline

    ____ Nardil

2. List two side effects associated with each of the following psychotherapeutic drugs.

    a. Phenothiazines:

    b. Tricyclic antidepressants:

    c. MAO inhibitors:

3. List at least five foods that are contraindicated for clients receiving MAO inhibitors.

4. Correctly name the extrapyramidal reactions pictured below.

a.

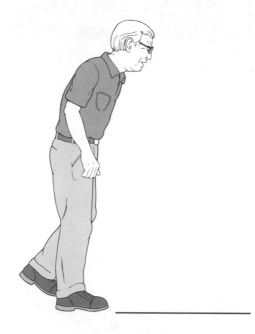

_____

b.

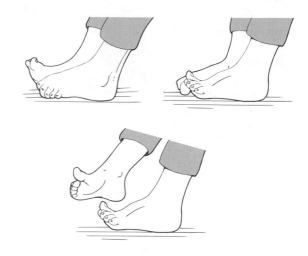

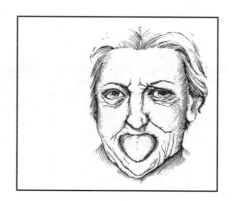

_____

c.

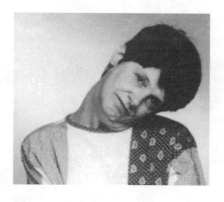

_____

d.

_____

Chapter 20   Overview of the Autonomic Nervous System

1. The simplest means by which the nervous system responds to environmental change is through the action of the _____.

2. Nerves that contain acetylcholine are called _____, and they are involved in _____.

3. The central nervous system's sensory input and motor output constitute a _____.

4. Muscarinic receptors are located in the _____.

5. Nicotinic receptors appear in the _____.

6. List the physiologic differences between the parasympathetic and the sympathetic nervous systems.

7. Match these terms and definitions commonly associated with the autonomic nervous system.

_____ Conduction   a. From one neuron to another neuron

_____ Neurohormonal transmission   b. On the postsynaptic effector cells

_____ Alpha 1 sites   c. On the presynaptic nerve terminals

_____ Alpha 2 sites   d. From a neuron to an effector organ

_____ Synaptic junction   e. Passage of a nerve impulse across a junction with the use of a chemical

_____ Neuroeffector junction   f. Passage of a nerve impulse along a nerve fiber or muscle fiber

Chapter 21   Drug Affecting the Parasympathetic Nervous System

1. Adrenergic blocking drugs block the action of the _____.

2. Cholinergic blocking drugs block the action of the _____.

3. Antimuscarinic drugs block the _____ and are also called _____ drugs.

4. Cholinergic drugs may be obtained from _____ or they may be _____. The two groups of cholinergic drugs available are _____ and _____.

5. The muscarinic effect is the action of _____ at the _____ nerve endings, which is like that of _____.

6. Describe the action of atropine.

7. List the uses of atropine.

8. List the important concepts to teach a client taking Nicorette.

9. Describe the steps the client should take in changing a nicotine transdermal patch.

10. Identify nursing diagnoses and interventions for a client receiving atropine systemically.

Chapter 22   Drugs Affecting the Sympathetic (Adrenergic) Nervous System

1. Match the physiologic response to the receptor stimulated.

    _____ Cardiac muscle   a. Alpha 1

    _____ Cerebral blood vessels   b. Alpha 2

    _____ Bronchial smooth muscle   c. Beta 1

    _____ Liver   d. Beta 2

    _____ Insulin secretion

    _____ Adipose tissue

    _____ Pupil size

    _____ Platelet aggregation

2. List the side effects of epinephrine.

3. Catecholamine produces a significant increase in cardiac contraction, or a positive _____ effect. It also increases heart rate, or a positive _____ effect. An increase in atrioventricular conduction, or a positive _____ effect, also occurs.

4. The alpha-adrenergic blocking agents fall into three categories: _____, _____, and _____.

5. List three drugs that interact with beta-adrenergic blocking agents and their physiologic effects.

1. Describe the basic disorder in Parkinson's disease, and list some of the signs and symptoms seen in the client.

2. List the main pharmacologic actions of antiparkinsonian agents.

3. List nursing interventions appropriate for a client receiving levodopa.

4. Describe myasthenia gravis.

5. List two drugs that interact with anticholinesterase agents and the effect that occurs.

6. List the more frequent side effects of the direct-acting skeletal muscle relaxant dantrolene.

7. Identify appropriate monitoring, intervention, and education strategies for a client receiving baclofen.

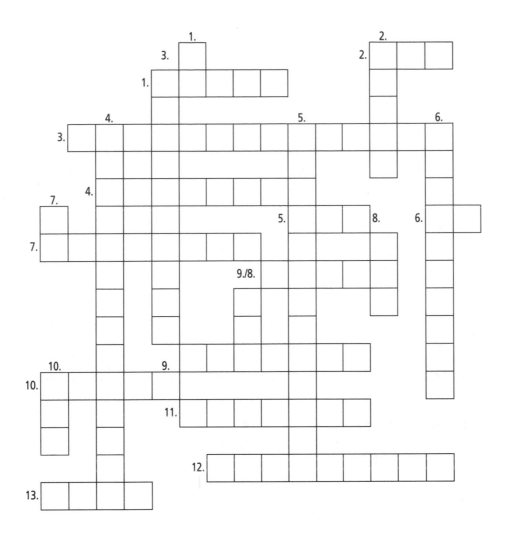

Across

1. Major parasympathetic nerve innervation of the heart
2. Abbreviation for adenosine triphosphatase
3. Name of law pertaining to force of heart contraction
4. Fibers that are part of conduction system of heart
5. Number of ventricles
6. Abbreviation for calcium
7. Term for speed
8. Term for when heart conduction does not occur
9. Term for the period of heart contraction
10. Organ that pumps blood
11. Main cation affecting electrical stimulation of the heart
12. Stimulus that changes the resting membrane
13. Calcium, potassium, and sodium are examples

Down

1. Abbreviation for sodium
2. Top chambers of the heart
3. Chambers that force blood to various parts of the body
4. Term for cardiac contraction recovery
5. Neurotransmitter that stimulates the vagus nerve
6. Digitalis is an example of this classification
7. Node that stimulates the heart to contract
8. Possible abbreviation for electrocardiogram
9. Letters on graph depicting ventricular contraction
10. Part of conduction system of heart

Chapter 25   Cardiac Glycosides

1. Word search:

AMRINONE   ECG   MILRINONE
CHF   FAB   NURSING
CHRONOTROPIC   FIBRILLATION   PACEMAKERS
DIGITALIZATION   GLYCOSIDE   SERUM
DIGOXIN   INOTROPIC   TOXICITY
DROMOTROPIC   LANOXIN

```
G  N  C  P  S  F  L  K  O  A  M  R  T  S  Q  D  W  V  K  X
Y  L  S  E  R  Z  Z  L  Q  W  H  F  O  Z  X  Z  H  V  I  K
O  S  R  W  E  J  G  K  P  J  A  B  X  W  C  L  B  Q  L  R
O  U  W  V  K  Y  X  U  A  C  V  L  I  E  R  H  P  E  S  R
M  B  P  X  A  H  A  Y  H  S  Q  Z  C  K  R  N  R  Z  I  U
R  Y  F  O  M  C  X  K  K  C  F  Z  I  G  J  B  J  Y  Z  V
J  I  F  E  E  W  J  W  R  M  J  A  T  L  X  Z  W  Z  W  V
F  H  A  O  C  E  D  X  H  B  G  L  Y  C  O  S  I  D  E  B
G  E  M  Y  A  H  W  A  L  V  E  C  R  H  D  L  B  M  I  Y
H  N  R  G  P  W  F  Z  G  Q  N  P  I  R  J  E  X  C  E  K
N  O  I  T  A  L  L  I  R  B  I  F  O  O  Z  V  C  M  N  O
U  N  N  S  O  A  F  D  G  Z  X  M  U  N  I  X  O  G  I  D
R  I  O  U  R  U  V  P  I  N  O  T  R  O  P  I  C  Y  H  J
K  R  N  V  R  U  U  J  M  T  N  A  P  T  X  R  T  D  Y  Z
T  L  E  S  P  N  N  F  R  D  A  J  E  R  Y  E  K  T  J  Q
Q  I  J  J  K  E  X  O  C  O  L  M  B  O  A  I  B  J  Y  O
X  M  Q  W  U  D  P  Y  O  N  G  F  A  P  Z  N  R  O  C  Q
G  M  N  R  R  I  D  I  G  I  T  A  L  I  Z  A  T  I  O  N
W  O  B  R  C  B  D  P  V  Q  Q  B  W  C  O  Z  X  B  Q  K
J  W  W  W  J  B  H  Y  J  U  Y  W  J  B  Y  X  J  Z  X  W
```

2. List the adverse reactions associated with digoxin.

3. List at least three factors that may predispose a client to digitalis toxicity.

4. Describe the client education strategies required for a client receiving cardiac glycoside therapy.

5. List nursing diagnoses for a client receiving amrinone.

1. Cryptoquote. The cryptoquote is a substitution cipher in which one letter stands for another. If you think Y equals A, then every Y in the sentence is an A. Look for one- or two-letter words to begin to decipher the sentence; then look for patterns of lettters until you solve the puzzle.

   Clue: A = D

   AHCWBHFBPOZ OC JZSCITA DH Z AOCIWATW ZLLTJBOUE FBT JTNNC IL FBT JIUASJFOIU CHCFTP IW FBT PHIJZWAOSP.

2. Match the antidysrhythmic drug to its classification.

   ____ procainamide   a. Group I-A

   ____ mexiletine   b. Group I-B

   ____ adenosine   c. Group I-C

   ____ quinidine   d. Group I

   ____ propranolol   e. Group II

   ____ Encainide   f. Group III

   ____ bretylium   g. Group IV

   ____ lidocaine

   ____ sotalol

   ____ moricizine

3. Indicate whether the following are true (**T**) or false (**F**).

   ____ Quinidine is used to help stop abnormally slow dysrhythmias and restore a normal sinus rhythm when persons have organic heart disease.

   ____ Quinidine depresses excitability, velocity of conduction, and contractility of the heart.

   ____ Propranolol is used primarily to speed heart rate in patients with bradyarrhythmias.

   ____ Lidocaine is not to be administered to patients with Adams-Stokes syndrome.

Chapter 27   Antihypertensives

1. Describe the renin-angiotensin-aldosterone mechanism.

2. To which antihypertensive agents do blacks generally respond better?

3. List the special needs of the older adult receiving antihypertensives.

4. Indicate whether the following are true **(T)** or false **(F)**.

_____ Vasodilators promote blood flow to the extremities by increasing the lumen of arterioles.

_____ Vasodilators act to decrease blood pressure.

_____ Flushing, sweating, nausea, vomiting, tingling, and headache may all be produced by peripheral vasodilating agents.

_____ Peripheral pulses should be taken routinely on a client receiving peripheral vasodilating agents.

5. Fill in the blanks for clonidine.

Routes		
Distribution		
Dosage		
Action		
Adverse effects		
Nursing diagnoses		

Chapter 28   Calcium Channel Blockers

1. In automaticity, a cell initiates _____.

2. Calcium channel blockers are used primarily for their _____, _____, and _____ properties.

3. Calcium channel blockers inhibit the contraction of smooth muscle of the peripheral arterioles, resulting in widespread reduction in _____ and _____.

4. List two drugs that interact with calcium channel blocking agents and their possible effects.

5. List the side effects of nifedipine.

6. List five education strategies for a client receiving a calcium channel blocker.

7. What is the treatment for bradycardia caused by an overdose of calcium blocker?

Chapter 29   Vasodilators and Antihemorrheologic Agents

1. Angina is characterized by _____; it occurs with _____ and is relieved by _____.

2. Nitrates are effective for the treatment of angina pectoris because of _____.

3. Carboxyhemoglobin is the presence of _____ in smokers, who have reduced amounts of _____.

4. Intermittent claudication is a syndrome that results from _____; it is characteristic of _____.

5. Indicate whether the following are true (**T**) or false (**F**).

    _____ The vasodilators have been very effective in treating peripheral occlusive arterial disease.

    _____ Headaches and hypotension may be caused by vasodilation of blood vessels affected by nitroglycerin.

    _____ Long-acting nitrates are used therapeutically to abort an acute attack of angina pectoris.

6. Identify client education strategies when administering buccal extended-release nitroglycerin.

7. List the three therapeutic objectives for the use of antianginal agents.

8. Describe the mechanism of action of pentoxifylline.

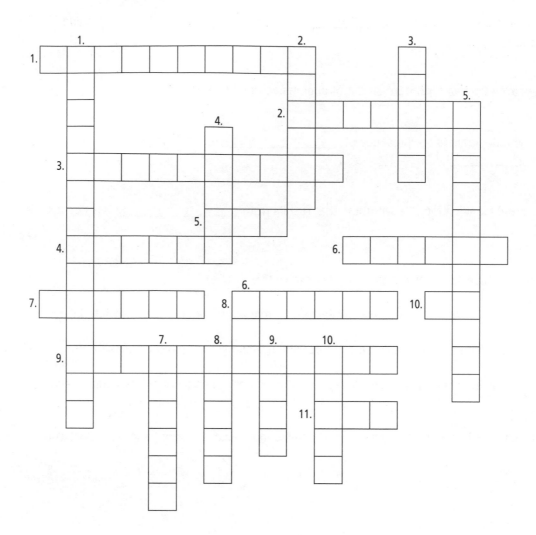

Across

1. Cells that fight infection
2. Protein that helps maintain osmolality
3. Combines with oxygen
4. Liquid portion of the blood
5. Abbreviation for hematocrit
6. Chemical substance involved with clotting
7. Combines with platelets to reinforce clots
8. Disorder caused by decreased hemoglobin
9. Another word for platelets
10. Antigen present on RBC
11. Abbreviation for platelet

Down

1. Hormone produced by kidney
2. Pooling of blood
3. Fluid other than blood that carries leukocytes
4. First letter of the Greek alphabet
5. One type of WBC
6. Types of blood
7. Gas carried by RBCs
8. Fluid that circulates in arteries and veins
9. Must occur to prevent hemorrhage
10. Various blood classifications

1. Match the anticoagulant agent to its route.

____ warfarin

____ anisindione

____ heparin

____ enoxaparin

____ danaparoid

____ dicumarol

a. Parenteral

b. Oral

2. Match the drug to the reaction it causes when given with oral anticoagulants.

____ Androgens

____ Estrogens

____ Vitamin K

____ Aspirin

____ cimetidine

____ Oral contraceptives

____ meperidine

____ Barbiturates

a. Increases effect of an anticoagulant

b. Decreases effect of an anticoagulant

3. List symptoms that may occur if a client is reacting to a blood transfusion.

4. Identify risks associated with coadministration of thrombolytics and anticoagulants.

5. Identify nursing implications for an older adult receiving anticoagulants.

Chapter 32   Antihyperlipidemic Drugs

1. Hyperlipidemia is a/an _____ disorder characterized by _____ and _____.

2. An important relationship exists between atherosclerosis and _____.

3. High-density lipoproteins pick up _____ from _____ and carry them to _____.

4. Lipoproteins are _____ bound to _____, which act as carriers; they are classified according to their _____.

5. Low-density lipoproteins contain the major portion of _____ in blood and may be considered _____.

6. Chylomicrons are the _____ particles and least _____ of the lipoproteins; they are produced in _____.

7. List two drugs that interact with bile acid sequestering agents and the effects they produce.

8. List education strategies appropriate for a client receiving clofibrate.

9. List side effects of reductase inhibitors.

1. Describe the major components of the urinary system.

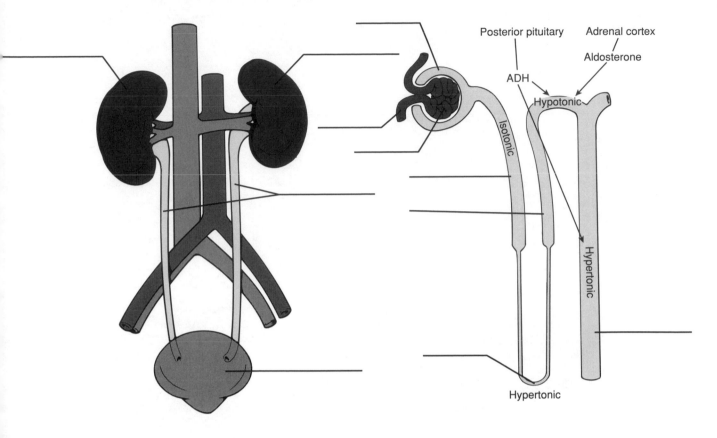

2. Match the function to the site of the nephron in which it occurs.

_____ Sodium reabsorption

_____ Chloride reabsorption

_____ Glucose reabsorption

_____ Urine concentration

_____ Aldosterone affects sodium reabsorption

_____ Increased potassium secretion

_____ Passive water uptake produces a hypertonic filtrate

_____ Passive sodium reabsorption produces a hypotonic filtrate

_____ Potassium reabsorbed

a. Proximal tubule

b. Distal tubule

c. Descending loop of Henle

d. Ascending loop of Henle

e. Collecting duct

3. Define:

   a. Hypertonic

   b. Hypotonic

Chapter 34   Diuretics

1. Match the diuretic to the site of the nephron it influences to produce therapeutic action.

_____ furosemide

_____ acetazolamide

_____ hydrochlorothiazide

_____ spironolactone

_____ Diamox

_____ bumetanide

a. Proximal tubule

b. Distal tubule

c. Loop of Henle

2. Diuretics are the most _____ used medications. They are useful in treating _____, _____, _____, and _____. They influence water and _____ balance. Their primary effect is on _____ function of the _____.

3. Match the sign or symptom to the electrolyte imbalance.

_____ Lethargy

_____ Twitching

_____ Weakness

_____ Irritability

_____ Seizures

_____ Diarrhea

_____ Abnormal ECG

_____ Flaccid paralysis

_____ Vomiting

a. Hypokalemia

b. Hyperkalemia

c. Hyponatremia

d. Hypocalcemia

4. List special nursing considerations when administering diuretics to an elderly client.

Chapter 35   Uricosuric Drugs

1. Gout is a/an _____ disease that manifests itself by attacks of _____, _____, and _____ of joints.

2. The hallmark of gout is _____, or high levels of _____.

3. Tophi are _____.

4. Xanthine oxidase is the _____.

5. List the treatment goals for gout.

6. Probenecid has another action not related to gout. Describe it.

7. Indicate whether the following are true (T) or false (F).

   _____ Allopurinol inhibits the production of uric acid.

   _____ Colchicine decreases phagocytosis and the motility of leukocytes.

   _____ Colchicine has no direct effect on the serum uric acid level.

   _____ Anticoagulants should not be given concurrently with allopurinol.

   _____ Alopecia is a frequent side effect of colchicine.

8. Develop an educational tool listing drugs that interact with probenecid to give to an older adult.

Chapter 36   Drug Therapy for Renal System Dysfunction

1. Acute renal failure, or a rapid _____ in renal function, occurs in approximately _____% of all hospitalized individuals.

2. Chronic renal failure is _____ impaired kidney function.

3. Azotemia is a build-up of _____.

4. End-stage renal disease leads to the need for _____, _____, or _____.

5. In peritoneal dialysis, needed _____ are passed into the bloodstream and _____ are removed, through the processes of _____, _____, and _____.

6. Identify two laboratory tests used to evaluate renal functioning.

7. List signs and symptoms that occur in a client with chronic renal failure (CRF).

8. Why is epoetin alfa given to a client with CRF?

9. Describe the two dosing methods used for clients with renal insufficiency or impairment.

10. Identify four drugs associated with renal toxicity or dysfunction and the specific toxic effects or dysfunction to which they are related.

11. Word search:

ACUTE
AZOTEMIA
BUN
CHRONIC
CREATININE
DIAGNOSIS
DOSING

DRUGS
EPOETIN
ERSD
EVALUATION
FAILURE
FLUID
HEMODIALYSIS

INTERVENTIONS
KIDNEY
NURSING
PERITONEAL
RENAL
WEIGHT

```
A C K S D A X E D Q Q Q R Y Y
S N O I T N E V R E T N I A E
T N W S D T E X Q F H G H H A
O G S Y A N Q J W K G K R P P
R X H L L A E N O T I R E P A
D Q L A N E R Y U K E W T L C
L G N I S R U N G K W B M N U
X R Z D A B K Q N L I F C T X
H Z X O E J R W Z T C I E E J
H N B M U A B F A I L U R E F
H B E E L U C H R O N I C L D
C D S H N M A U D E V D U H C
T R G A E A Z O T E M I A T R
B N X C M R S D P E D A W V E
F A K C P I S O B U B G M S A
O P N X N L E D Y P Y N X G T
Y X B G E T Y Q R D P O G Q I
G S Q V I H R O D U D S R Z N
V M C N D T T V N U G I O A I
V G F R A R E Z D C O S T U N
U X Q N O I T A U L A V E S E
```

1. Draw arrows to explain how diffusion affects internal and external respiration.

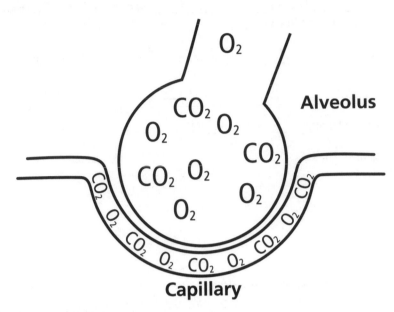

2. List factors determining airway efficiency

3. Describe the effect of the autonomic nervous system on respiration.

4. Describe elements of central control of respiration.

Chapter 38   Mucokinetic, Bronchodilator, and Antiasthmatic Drugs

1. Mucokinetic agents promote the removal of _____ and prevent _____.

2. Sputum, or _____, is a/an _____ secretion that is a production of _____; it consists mainly of _____.

3. Aerosol therapy is a form of _____ treatment; it is delivered through _____.

4. Mucolytics, also called _____, exert a/an _____ effect on mucus.

5. Bronchodilators are used to treat _____.

6. List actions of xanthine derivatives.

7. List the effects of aerosol therapy on the respiratory system.

8. List nursing interventions for a client when acetylcysteine is administered for its antidotal use.

9. Contrast the old and the current methods of classifying asthma.

10. List the side effects/adverse reactions of epinephrine.

11. List education strategies for client learning how to use an inhaler.

12. Indicate whether the following are true (**T**) or false (**F**).

_____ The effectiveness of the methylxanthines depends on their conversion to theophylline.

_____ The rate of absorption of oral theophylline depends on the dosage form used.

_____ Xanthine derivatives relax smooth muscle and cardiac muscle.

13. List the strategies for reducing or eliminating environmental allergens.

1. Pulse oximetry provides a continuous reading of _____.

2. Diminished oxygen tension in the blood is known as _____.

3. Of all the tissues affected by _____, or oxygen lack, the _____ is the most susceptible to disruption of normal function and irreversible damage.

4. Individuals with _____ are subject to _____, which is high carbon dioxide content in the blood.

5. Dyspnea is _____ and may indicate the need for _____.

6. Oxygen is a/an _____, _____, and _____ gas that is essential for _____.

7. Carbon dioxide is a/an _____, _____ gas; when used as a pharmacologic agent it affects _____, _____, and _____.

8. Identify seven methods of oxygen administration.

9. Identify learning needs of clients receiving antihistamines.

10. Indicate whether the following are true (T) or false (F).

_____ If a narcotic antitussive agent is given with a CNS depressant, a reduced dosage should be used.

_____ Antitussives are often given in chronic pulmonary disease.

_____ The amount of narcotic in antitussive products is very small, and there is almost no risk of producing drug dependence in a client.

_____ All antihistamines are available over the counter.

_____ Antihistamines are relatively safe and most clients will not have trouble with them.

Chapter 40   Overview of the Gastrointestinal Tract

1. Food substances entering the alimentary canal undergo _____ and _____ changes called _____.

2. Deglutition is also called _____.

3. Difficulty in swallowing is known as _____.

4. The peristaltic process is the squeezing of the _____ down the _____; it is accomplished by _____.

5. Cholecystitis is _____; it is often associated with the presence of _____.

6. The alimentary canal extends from the _____ to the _____.

7. Match the disorder/disease to the anatomic site in the GI system.

_____ Gingivitis	a. Mouth
_____ Gastritis	b. Esophagus
_____ Achalasia	c. Stomach
_____ Hepatitis	d. Small intestine
_____ Malabsorption	e. Large intestine
_____ Diabetes	f. Liver
_____ Diverticulitis	g. Gallbladder
_____ Peptic ulcer	h. Pancreas
_____ Colitis	
_____ Cholelithiasis	
_____ Constipation	
_____ Hemorrhoids	

8. Describe how the autonomic nervous system affects the GI system.

Chapter 41   Drugs Affecting the Gastrointestinal Tract

1. Indicate the actions of antacids and H$_2$ receptor antagonists by putting **A** (antacids); **H** (H$_2$ receptor antagonists); **B** (both); or **N** (neither) in front of the following possible actions.

_____ Neutralize hydrochloric acid

_____ Increase gastric pH

_____ Buffer hydrochloric acid

_____ Inhibit secretion of gastric acid

_____ Decrease gastric pH

_____ Promote healing of gastric and duodenal ulcers

2. What information would be important to tell a parent who is using a mouthwash containing alcohol?

3. Match the antiemetic with its proposed site of action.

_____ diazepam

_____ diphenidol

_____ antihistamines

_____ anticholinergics

_____ phenothiazine

a. Emetic center

b. Chemoreceptor trigger zone

c. Cerebral cortex

d. Peripheral sites

4. List nursing interventions appropriate for a client receiving metoclopramide.

5. List the most frequent side effects of ondansetron.

6. Describe *Helicobacter pylori* and its role in peptic ulcer disease.

7. Develop a teaching plan for an elderly client receiving famotidine.

8. Describe how proton pump inhibitors exert their therapeutic effect.

9. List nursing diagnoses for a client receiving chenodiol.

10. List foods a nurse can recommend to prevent or to treat constipation.

11. Suggest nursing diagnoses for use of antidiarrheals and appropriate nursing interventions.

Chapter 42   Overview of the Eye

1. The eye is the _____ organ for the sense of _____ .

2. The cornea is the _____ covering of the eye; it is normally _____ , so it allows_____ to enter the eye.

3. Contraction of the sphincter muscle causes _____ of the pupil, or _____ .

4. Contraction of the dilator muscle causes _____ of the pupil, or _____ .

5. Accommodation occurs when the lens _____ , which ensures that the image on the retina is _____ .

6. With age the lens may lose its _____ and become _____ ; this is known as _____ .

7. Define cycloplegia.

8. Describe how miotic drugs affect the eye.

9. Describe how mydriatic drugs affect the eye.

10. Identify the function of the aqueous humor.

11. Identify the factors affecting accommodation.

12. Identify two structures within the retina that act as visual receptors.

13. Name the four protective mechanisms of the eye.

Chapter 43   Ophthalmic Drugs

1. Glaucoma is characterized by _____; it can lead to _____.

2. Miotics are useful in treating _____ and _____.

3. Anticholinesterase drugs inhibit _____ by _____.

4. Define the following terms.

   Conjunctivitis _____

   Hordeolum _____

   Chalazion _____

   Keratitis _____

   Uveitis _____

5. List the three major types of glaucoma.

6. List four possible nursing diagnoses for a client receiving ophthalmic drugs.

7. List five systemic drugs and their effects on the eye.

8. Describe how to instill eyedrops and eye ointments in children and adults.

9. Identify adverse systemic effects from beta-blocking antiglaucoma agents.

Chapter 44   Overview of the Ear

1. The tympanic membrane is a/an _____ located between the _____ and
_____.

2. The eustachian tube connects the _____ and the _____; it is usually collapsed
except when _____.

3. The auditory ossicles are the _____, _____, and _____; the ossicles amplify and transmit _____.

4. The primary organ of hearing is the _____.

5. List the anatomic parts of the three divisions of the ear.

    External ear:

    Middle ear:

    Inner ear:

6. Explain the function of the eustachian tube.

7. Name the middle ear infection most often reported in children.

8. Match the ear disorder to its anatomic site.

    _____ Seborrhea   a. External ear

    _____ Otosclerosis   b. Middle ear

    _____ Otitis media   c. Inner ear

    _____ Tympanic perforation

    _____ Meniere's disease

1. State the side effects of chloramphenicol.

2. Describe how to administer ear drops, suggesting differences in administration for adult and pediatric clients.

3. List monitoring, intervention, and education strategies for a client receiving a drug that induces ototoxicity.

4. List the use(s) of the following OTC otic drugs:

    Auro Ear Drops

    Aurocaine Drops

    Earsol-HC Drops

5. List five drugs that can lead to ototoxicity.

1. Fill in the various endocrine glands on the following picture.

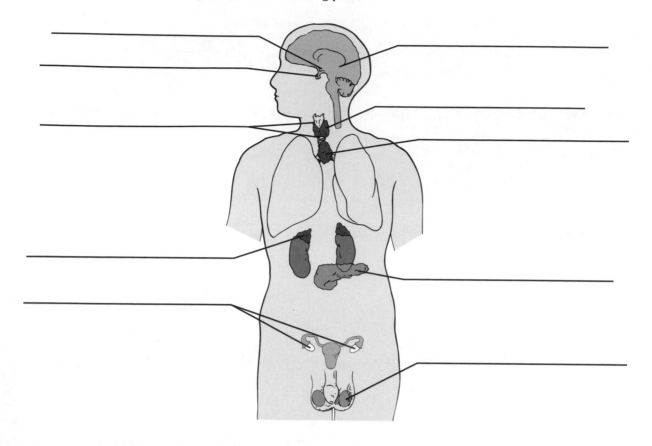

2. List the vital physiologic processes that hormones affect.

3. Match the hormone with the gland it is secreted from.

_____ MSH

_____ Aldosterone

_____ PTH

_____ STH

_____ LH

_____ Vasopressin

_____ Insulin

_____ Glucocorticoid

_____ Androgens

_____ Triiodothyronine

_____ ACTH

_____ Glucagon

_____ Oxytocin

a. Anterior pituitary

b. Posterior pituitary

c. Thyroid

d. Parathyroid

e. Adrenal

f. Pancreas

1. Word search:

ABUSE
ACTH
ALLERGIC
ANTERIOR
CONFUSION
CRH
DIABETES
DWARFISM
ELECTROLYTES

ENDOCRINE
GIGANTISM
GONADOTROPIN
HORMONE
HUMATROPE
INSIPIDUS
LH
NURSING

PITUITARY
POSTERIOR
SOMATOSTATIN
SOMATREM
TRH
TSH
URINE
VASOPRESSIN

```
E  A  A  N  T  E  R  I  O  R  C  C  J  M  R  I  Y  I  H
L  C  M  B  P  R  W  O  S  A  O  D  P  K  I  X  P  L  U
E  T  J  I  U  C  H  Q  L  N  D  I  O  U  N  X  I  M  M
C  H  S  T  E  S  W  L  F  K  W  A  S  L  S  V  T  E  A
T  O  F  T  L  Y  E  U  J  K  A  B  T  S  I  E  U  R  T
R  R  V  N  F  R  S  Q  U  R  R  E  E  O  P  I  I  T  R
O  M  H  P  G  I  U  L  K  I  F  T  R  M  I  X  T  A  O
L  O  R  I  O  I  S  C  R  S  I  E  I  A  D  V  A  M  P
Y  N  C  N  F  M  Z  C  H  J  S  S  O  T  U  R  R  O  E
T  E  N  I  R  C  O  D  N  E  M  J  R  O  S  M  Y  S  F
E  B  S  G  I  G  A  N  T  I  S  M  L  S  L  Z  R  M  X
S  N  U  R  S  I  N  G  O  N  A  D  O  T  R  O  P  I  N
E  N  I  S  S  E  R  P  O  S  A  V  O  A  C  K  J  M  F
K  X  G  R  K  W  U  B  Y  A  N  X  V  T  H  C  W  Q  O
W  E  X  Z  U  S  A  T  T  I  E  J  N  I  R  J  M  X  X
D  I  C  X  D  S  I  C  G  P  V  Y  E  N  A  A  X  M  O
```

2. List the side effects of vasopressin.

3. Suggest monitoring, intervention, and education strategies for a child receiving somatrem.

4. In addition to the drug's adverse effects, what risks face athletes who abuse growth hormone?

Chapter 48   Drugs Affecting the Parathyroid and Thyroid

1. Adenomas are tumors often seen in _____.

2. Desiccated thyroid is used for _____.

3. Iodine is the oldest of the _____ drugs; it inhibits _____.

4. Myxedema is a form of _____.

5. RAI, or _____, is preferred for _____.

6. Match the sign or symptom to the endocrine disorder.

_____ Diarrhea   a. Hyperthyroidism

_____ Renal stones   b. Hypothyroidism

_____ Brittle hair   c. Hyperparathyroidism

_____ Fast reflexes   d. Hypoparathyroidism

_____ Irritability

_____ Calcium level decreased

_____ Ptosis

_____ Lethargic

_____ Cold, dry skin

_____ Bone pain

_____ Intolerance to heat

7. List two medications used to increase serum calcium levels in clients with hypoparathyroidism.

8. List two diagnostic agents used to assess thyroid function.

9. Identify the education needs of a client receiving sodium iodide ^{131}I.

1. Corticosteroids are adrenocortical _____ that are divided into two classes, _____ and _____.

2. Circadian rhythm is based on a/an _____ cycle and appears to be controlled by the _____.

3. Ultradian rhythms are _____ functions with frequencies greater than _____.

4. In the fight-or-flight phenomenon, _____ are suddenly released; they increase _____ to provide energy for _____.

5. List three actions of glucocorticoids.

6. List at least one adverse effect of adrenocorticoids as they affect the following body systems:

   Gastrointestinal

   Immune

   Musculoskeletal

7. Identify two drugs that interact with mineralocorticoids and their effects.

8. List assessment information important to obtain in a client receiving aminoglutethimide.

Chapter 50   Drugs Affecting the Pancreas

1. The two primary hormones released by the pancreas are _____ and _____.

2. The process in which the liver breaks down and releases its glucose stores is called _____; the production of glucose is called _____.

3. Outline the instructions for a client using intrasite rotation of insulin injection sites.

4. List five "quick fixes" for clients with mild hypoglycemia.

5. Describe how oral hypoglycemic agents lower blood glucose.

6. List special nursing interventions related to insulin administration.

7. Match the sign or symptom to the blood glucose disorder.

_____ Cold sweating   a. Hyperglycemia

_____ Thirst   b. Hypoglycemia

_____ Polyuria

_____ Pallor

_____ Blurred vision

_____ Anxiety

_____ Fruity breath

8. Describe the relationship of glucagon to the regulation of blood glucose with hypoglycemia.

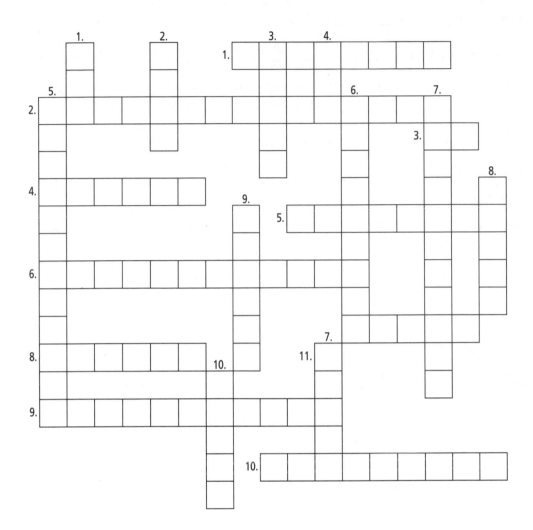

Across

1. Forms on ovary and releases ovum
2. Part of autonomic nervous system controlling orgasm
3. Abbreviation for luteinizing hormone
4. Garnete-producing gland
5. Common site for cancer in older men
6. Male hormone
7. Meaning "seed"
8. Pleasurable end to sexual act
9. Release of semen
10. Cutting of vas deferens

Down

1. Egg
2. Abbreviation of interstitial cell-stimulating hormone
3. Gland which releases ova
4. Abbreviation for luteotropic hormone
5. Female hormone increased in pregnancy
6. Female hormones
7. Male "menopause"
8. Fluid containing sperm
9. Womb
10. Folds of skin at opening of vagina
11. Erectile organ of the male

Chapter 52 Drugs Affecting Women's Health and the Female Reproductive System

1. Gonadorelin is a/an _____; it stimulates _____.

2. Monophasic oral contraception is _____; it is the _____ commonly used.

3. Biphasic oral contraception supplies low levels of hormones in the _____ phase, which is increased during the _____ phase of the menstrual cycle.

4. Triphasic oral contraception most closely simulates _____.

5. Anovulation is the absence of _____; it is a suspected pathologic condition in individuals with _____.

6. Indicate which of the following symptoms are adverse effects (**A**) and which are contraindications (**C**) to use of oral birth control pills.

_____ Coronary artery disease   _____ Pregnancy

_____ Weight gain   _____ Acne

_____ Breast tenderness   _____ Decreased menses

_____ Nausea   _____ Abdominal bloating

_____ Tiredness   _____ Hot flashes

_____ Depression   _____ High blood pressure

7. List learning needs for a client receiving Clomid.

Chapter 53   Drugs for Labor and Delivery

1. Oxytocics stimulate _____, resulting in _____.

2. Preterm labor is _____; it occurs in approximately _____% of all pregnancies.

3. Multiparity is defined as _____.

4. List the side effects of Ergotrate.

5. State how terbutaline is used in labor and delivery.

6. What safety factors are taught to the client using terbutaline at home?

7. Identify possible nursing diagnoses for a pregnant client receiving ritodrine for premature labor.

1. Word search:

ANDROGENS	ERECTIONS	NURSING
ANEMIA	FINASTERIDE	PROSTATE
ANTINEOPLASTIC	GYNECOMASTIA	PROTEIN
ASSESSMENT	HYPOGONADISM	PUBERTY
BPH	INDICATIONS	REACTIONS
CANCER	JAUNDICE	SAW
DEPRESSION	LIBIDO	TESTOSTERONE
DIZZINESS		

```
U  T  K  P  N  I  I  B  G  E  G  C  C  O  D  I  B  I  L
T  B  A  V  R  R  D  P  F  N  E  I  U  Y  V  L  S  W  Y
P  S  S  R  G  G  Z  H  C  C  I  T  F  Q  F  B  S  W  O
T  Q  J  Z  C  R  H  M  N  A  S  S  E  S  S  M  E  N  T
H  A  C  F  N  O  E  K  U  P  E  A  R  N  S  L  N  A  M
T  Q  H  S  L  Y  V  C  U  I  D  L  W  U  H  Q  I  A  D
V  R  A  B  P  L  Z  B  P  N  I  P  J  Q  N  F  Z  I  E
J  C  F  D  R  M  E  A  N  D  R  O  G  E  N  S  Z  T  P
L  U  C  J  O  R  L  N  A  I  E  E  E  K  H  M  I  S  R
E  P  D  H  T  M  L  E  Y  C  T  N  C  Z  R  E  D  A  E
M  R  O  Y  E  X  M  M  S  A  S  I  I  N  E  R  J  M  S
I  O  N  N  I  Q  X  I  P  T  A  T  D  P  A  E  Q  O  S
D  S  T  I  N  D  Q  A  C  I  N  N  N  U  C  C  X  C  I
W  T  Y  H  V  J  S  U  X  O  I  A  U  R  T  T  S  E  O
O  A  X  S  D  B  T  T  Z  N  F  O  A  R  I  I  X  N  N
Y  T  B  L  D  D  O  X  V  S  C  U  J  N  O  O  V  Y  K
T  E  S  T  O  S  T  E  R  O  N  E  I  X  N  N  A  G  O
F  U  J  A  I  A  M  P  Y  R  S  D  B  G  S  S  Q  Y  K
O  V  O  U  Z  O  O  H  Y  P  O  G  O  N  A  D  I  S  M
```

2. List uses for testosterone.

3. List two drugs that interact with testosterone and their effects.

4. Identify possible nursing diagnoses for a male client receiving testosterone.

5. BPH, or _____, is hypertrophy of _____.

6. List the side effects/adverse reactions of finasteride.

Chapter 55   Drugs Affecting Sexual Behavior

1. Libido is known as _____.

2. Oozing of a fluid through pores is called _____.

3. Impotence is the inability of a man to _____ or _____ an erection.

4. Variations in female hormones may produce the _____, _____, and _____ associated with PMS, or _____.

5. Hypersexuality is abnormally increased _____ and _____.

6. List three drugs that impair sexual behavior and the probable action.

7. Describe the nursing goals in dealing with human sexuality.

Chapter 56   Principles of Antineoplastic Chemotherapy

1. Cancer is a _____ term that includes _____; cancer is second to _____ as a cause of death.

2. Spread of cancer is called _____.

3. The Pap smear is a/an _____ test capable of detecting _____.

4. Dose-limiting effects are _____ reactions that indicate that _____ and _____.

5. Describe gompertzian growth.

6. Describe what happens in each cell cycle phase:

   G1 phase

   S phase

   G2 phase

   M phase

7. In addition to affecting malignant cells, antineoplastic agents commonly affect some normal cells in the body. Fill in the following chart with the adverse effect most likely to be produced by the affected cells.

	Normal cells affected	Adverse response
GI tract		
Bone marrow		
Hair follicles		
Mouth		

8. Propose a nursing intervention for each of the following side effects:

   Constipation

   Alopecia

   Stomatitis

9. At home, how should the client or caregiver handle soiled bedpans and containers contaminated with vomitus?

Chapter 57　　Antineoplastic Chemotherapy Agents

1. Antineoplastic agents act by _____.

2. Although antimetabolites have a structure similar to _____, they interfere with _____.

3. Alkylating agents substitute _____ for _____ in DNA.

4. Antibiotic antitumor agents interfere with _____ by _____.

5. Mitotic inhibitors are _____ that block _____.

6. "Leucovorin rescue" describes treatments that use leucovorin to reduce _____.

7. Fill in the following chart associating antineoplastic drug actions with applicable drug.

Antineoplastic drug	Action
	Interferes with synthesis of DNA and RNA
	Prevents cell division and protein synthesis
	Binds DNA and inhibits RNA synthesis
	Inhibits mitosis during M-phase
	Inhibits virus replication, decreases cell proliferation, and enhances phagocyte activity
	Produces stable microtubule bundles and interferes with the late G-2 mitotic phase in cell cycle

8. Match the side effect/adverse reaction to the specific antineoplastic drug.

____ Dark discoloration of skin and fingernails　　a. cisplatin

____ Tinnitus　　b. 5-FU

____ Chills　　c. Cytoxan

____ Paresthesias of hands and feet　　d. vincristine

9. Describe antidote administration for doxorubicin.

1. Fill in the blanks describing the body temperature control mechanism.

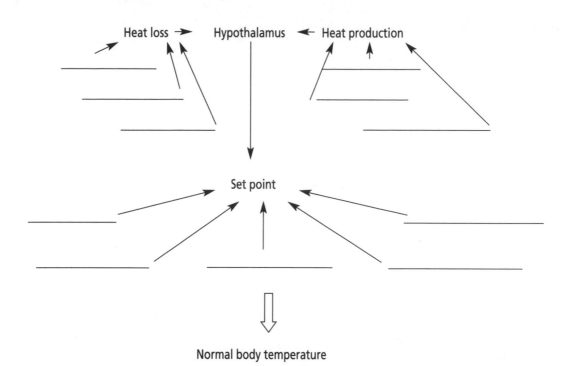

2. Match the antimicrobial to its mechanism of action.

____ sulfonamide

____ erythromycin

____ penicillin

____ amphotericin B

____ rifampin

____ tetracycline

____ INH

____ vancomycin

a. Inhibits cell wall synthesis

b. Alters membrane permeability

c. Antimetabolite

d. Inhibits protein synthesis

3. Develop an education plan for a client receiving an antimicrobial.

Chapter 59   Antibiotics

1. Antibiotics are substances that _____ or _____ the growth of
   _____; the four major classifications of antibiotics are _____,
   _____, _____, and _____.

2. The most effective and least toxic of the available antimicrobial drugs are the _____.

3. Identify on the following figure the area indicating the therapeutic range, the area that represents the trough, and the area that represents the peak.

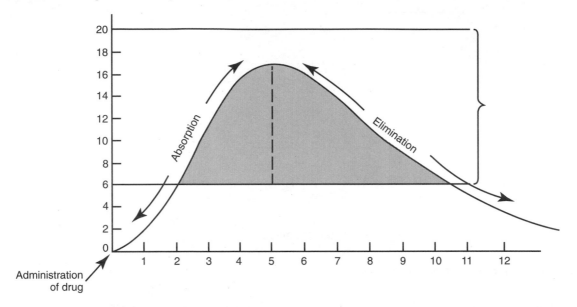

4. Describe the relationship and the importance of the peak and trough levels in clients receiving antibiotics.

5. Fill in the following table with the side effects to monitor with the specific antibiotic.

Antibiotic	Side effects to monitor
Chloramphenicol	
Erythromycin	
Clindamycin	
Ciprofloxacin	
Lincomycin	
Vancomycin	

6. Indicate whether the following are true **(T)** or false **(F)**.

_____ Drug interactions with antibiotics are common.

_____ All antibiotics should be taken with food or milk to decrease GI upset.

_____ Antibiotics rarely interfere with serum laboratory tests.

7. Discuss the needs of the pediatric client receiving antibiotics.

Chapter 60   Antifungal and Antiviral Drugs

1. Candidiasis is usually caused by _____; it is characterized by _____ , _____ , _____ , and _____.

2. Fungi are _____, _____ microorganisms.

3. Mycoses are _____ caused by _____.

4. The use of antimicrobial drugs before disease appears is called _____.

5. List important education strategies for a client receiving amphotericin B.

6. Describe the action of antiviral drugs.

7. List three drugs that interact with amantadine and their effects.

8. List side effects/adverse reactions of zidovudine.

9. List intervention strategies for administering didanosine tablets.

1. Word search:

AMEBIASIS   ERYTHROCYTIC   PINWORMS
AMINOSALICYLATE   GRANULOMATOUS   PREGNANCY
CBC   HANSEN   PYRAZINAMIDE
CHILDREN   HELMINTHS   RIFAMPIN
CHLOROQUINE   MALARIA   SAFETY
COMMUNITY   NURSING   TOXOPLASMOSIS
DISEASE   PARASITE   TRICHOMONIASIS
EDUCATION   PATHOGENESIS   TUBERCULOSIS

```
D J G R U H D S I S O L U C R E B U T Y
L W N X D D G I P A T H O G E N E S I S
I M I H R Y P F Z R M P I T G I R S G X
Y K S W V D Y X M A L A R I A P V I T Z
O Y R V J V T L W T I R C A F M E S O X
L T U E T I S A R A P N E P U A D A X L
A E N I U Q O R O L H C O Y R F I I O F
M F O E R Y T H R O C Y T I C I M N P O
E A T R C O M M U N I T Y O N R A O L W
B S F N P H Y D D G E C E R S S N M A O
I M L B V N I H A B B F C H P E I O S U
A M I N O S A L I C Y L A T E Y Z H M X
S I L Y E N D P D U H Q E S Q J A C O T
I F Y A S K U L Z R C T L G D P R I S B
S U S E E Z C Q P R E G N A N C Y R I T
G E N E D U C A T I O N K A U R P T S K
J A S U O T A M O L U N A R G S M F A K
H E L M I N T H S M R O W N I P L N D V
D L D W L T S K S G V Q S A T E D B B Q
Q O G F V L J Y K J F O B L J G Z K G B
```

2. Explain the life cycle of the malarial parasite.

3. Discuss transmission of the tubercle bacilli and nursing interventions to prevent the spread of tuberculosis.

4. What are the three medication management strategies for managing the tuberculosis client at home?

5. List the learning needs of a client receiving isoniazid.

6. List side effects of piperazine.

Chapter 62   Overview of the Immunologic System

1. Match the cells/tissues of the immune system to their major function. There may be more than one choice.

_____ IgG

_____ Thymus

_____ IgM

_____ T-helper

_____ Spleen

_____ T-cytotoxic

_____ IgE

_____ Tonsils

_____ IgD

_____ T-memory

a. Organs of immunity

b. Cell-mediated immunity

c. Humoral immunity

d. Antibodies

2. The complement system is a series of proteins that _____; when an antigen-antibody complex triggers complement, each component is _____.

3. Describe the actions of the following:

   IgG

   IgE

   IgD

   IgM

   IgA

4. Compare/contrast active immunity and passive immunity, including sources, effectiveness, methods, time to develop, duration, ease of reactivation, and purpose.

Chapter 63   Serums, Vaccines, and Other Immunizing Agents

1. Antibody titer is a measurement of _____; it can be useful in determining _____.

2. DPT refers to _____.

3. TOPV refers to _____.

4. MMR refers to _____.

5. Immunoprophylaxis is also called _____.

6. Discuss two current developments in immunization therapy.

7. List learning needs of parents of a child receiving immunizations.

8. Identify each vaccine as either active (**A**) or passive (**P**) immunity.

_____ Varicella-zoster

_____ Botulism antitoxin

_____ Cholera

_____ Influenza

_____ Hepatitis B immune globulin

_____ Rabies

_____ Measles immune globulin

_____ *Hemophilus* influenza

_____ Diphtheria antitoxin

_____ Typhoid

_____ Rho (D) immune globulin

_____ Polio

Chapter 64   Immunosuppressants and Immunomodulators

1. Immunosuppressant agents _____ or _____ an immune response; the primary immunosuppressant drugs are _____, _____, and _____.

2. SCIDS refers to _____.

3. In an immunocompromised state, the ability of the immune system is _____.

4. HIV refers to _____; it is the etiologic agent in _____.

5. Immunomodulating agents can activate _____ or modify _____.

6. Describe how HIV causes immunodeficiency.

7. List the most frequently reported side effects of cyclosporine.

8. Identify four criteria to include in an education plan for an immunosuppressed client.

9. List five clinical conditions that are indicators of AIDS in the patient with HIV.

Chapter 65   Overview of the Integumentary System

1. Identify the anatomic structures of the skin.

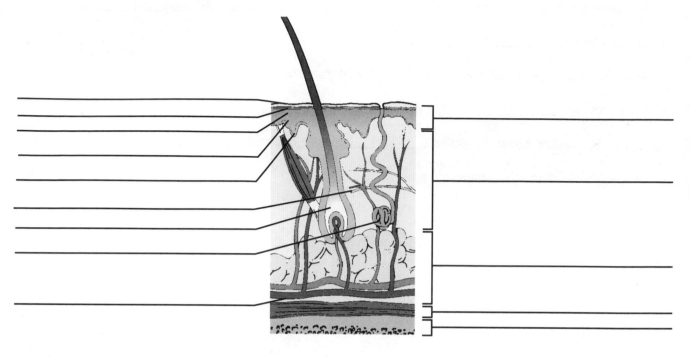

2. List the exocrine glands.

3. What is the normal pH of the skin?

4. List and describe the functions of the skin.

82

Chapter 66 Dermatologic Drugs

1. Match the description or example to the type of lesion.

_____ Raised, 1-2 cm diameter   a. Macule

_____ Herpes   b. Nodule

_____ Melanoma   c. Papule

_____ Lipomas   d. Plaques

_____ Flat, vary in color   e. Vesicle

_____ Psoriasis   f. Wheals

_____ Raised, irregular shape

_____ Acne

_____ Freckles

_____ Raised, less than 1 cm diameter

_____ Deep in dermis

_____ Urticaria

_____ Raised, fluid-filled

_____ Burns

_____ Raised, hard, rough

_____ Scabies

_____ Atopic dermatitis

2. List various forms of skin preparations.

3. Identify nursing diagnoses pertinent for a client receiving dermatologic agent therapy.

1. Cryptoquote. The cryptoquote is a substitution cipher in which one letter stands for another. If you think Y equals A, then every Y in the sentence is an A. Look for one- or two-letter words to begin to decipher the sentence; then look for patterns of letters until you solve the puzzle.

   Clue: Q = U

   APEF HPQKUK HKEZIOQZU ZK WUHQOGZQK QJHUIK.

2. Identify side effects of proteolytic enzyme preparations.

3. List the stages of decubitus ulcers and identify treatment modalities for each stage.

4. Describe several nursing strategies in prevention and treatment of pressure sores.

Chapter 68   Vitamins and Minerals

1. Vitamin supplement therapy may be essential during periods of _____, such as _____, _____, _____, and _____.

2. Vitamin deficiency is called _____.

3. Ascorbic acid is also known as _____.

4. Vitamins are classified according to their solubility. Which vitamins are fat soluble?

5. While vitamins have been given a letter of the alphabet to identify them, they all have one or more scientific names, depending on the number of chemicals making up that vitamin category. Fill in the following chart with the proper names of the vitamins.

Vitamin	Other names or chemical names
A	
B_1	
B_2	
B_3	
B_6	
B_9	
B_{12}	
C	
D	
E	

6. What is RDA?

7. Develop an education plan for a client receiving iron.

1. Match the symptoms at the left to the electrolyte imbalance (there may be more than one correct answer).

_____Lethargy   a. Hypocalcemia

_____Weakness   b. Hypermagnesemia

_____Peaked T waves   c. Hyponatremia

_____Tetany   d. Hyperkalemia

_____Flushing   e. Hypercalcemia

_____Athetoid movements   f. Hypokalemia

_____Amnesia   g. Hypomagnesemia

_____Paralysis   h. Hypernatremia

_____Seizures

_____Oliguria

2. List the intracellular electrolytes.

3. List the extracellular electrolytes.

4. Give an example of each type of solution and explain why it is used in each of the following categories.

Category	Solution	Use
Hydrating solution		
Isotonic solution		
Maintenance solution		

5. Match the sign or symptom to the type of dehydration associated with it.

_____ Thirst

_____ Increased ICF

_____ Shock

_____ Confusion

_____ Dry, furrowed tongue

_____ Low sodium

_____ Irritability

_____ Regular pulse

a. Isotonic

b. Hypotonic

c. Hypertonic

6. Until safer equipment is available, how can nurses protect their clients from the hazard of overdosing with electronic infusion devices?

Chapter 70   Enteral and Parenteral Nutrition

1. Enteral nutrition is _____ or _____ feeding, usually via a/an _____, _____, _____, _____, or _____ tube.

2. Hyperalimentation, also called _____, is the _____ approach to _____.

3. Amino acids are essential to _____, _____, and _____.

4. Essential amino acids cannot be _____.

5. List the drug and nutrient interactions that can occur with enteral nutrition therapy.

6. List several important data the nurse should assess in a client receiving TPN.

7. Identify several significant nursing education needs for a client receiving tube feedings.

8. Identify complications of parenteral nutrition arising from infection and sepsis.

Chapter 71   Antiseptics, Disinfectants, and Sterilants

1. Nosocomial infections are acquired in _____; the majority are _____ infections and _____ infections.

2. Medical asepsis, the absence of _____, and surgical asepsis, the absence of _____, are used to _____.

3. Sterilization destroys _____ on _____, in _____, or within _____; _____ cannot be sterilized.

4. Disinfectants are used only on _____; antiseptics are typically applied only to _____, so they must be _____ or made _____.

5. Identify the most effective measure to control the spread of infection.

6. Describe the action of antiseptics and disinfectants.

7. State uses of iodine compounds.

8. Identify nursing interventions for using iodine compounds.

9. List nursing considerations when using oxidizing agents.

1. Word search:

ANERGY   ANTIHISTAMINES   CHOLANGIOGRAPHY   CONTRAST
DETECTION   DIAGNOSTICS   EPINEPHRINE   FLUSHING
FUNCTIONING   IMMUNOSUPPRESSED   INDICATIONS   MRI
NURSING   ORGANS   RADIOACTIVE   RADIONUCLIDES
RADIOPAQUE   RADIOPHARMACEUTICAL   ROENTGEN   SCREENING
TOMOGRAPHY   TREATMENT   TUMORS   ULTRASONOGRAPHY
VISUALIZATION

```
S N O I T A C I D N I G L R B E G G N G H
D E S S E R P P U S O N U M M I C N N I U
L R U M B F N E G T N E O R T F Q I D U U
S G P S X Y V T D C M Y I C H A X N Q Y L
M X O C F Y Z A A O T H Z W G F J O B D T
I M K R Q Z B W N N R P Z N K R R I E D R
R L N E C R V X T T E A Y N J G V T M I A
P A Y E B N Q V I R A R R B A B E C B A S
R T D N X X T D H A T G G N U C P N F G O
A O S I W U M W I S M O S Y T E I U L N N
D M R N O Z M D S T E I R I I A N F U O O
I O T G U A M R T C N G O L K D E H S S G
O G C W T R C V A N T N M D A F P I H T R
N R N B V Y S T M D V A U J K F H T I I A
U A S U S A G I I T I L T C S S R W N C P
C P I B X Q G W N V L O N G H X I U G S H
L H N X S D R R E G E H P Y J X N Q E A Y
I Y G F S R F K S O F C C A Z A E R P J H
D A Q E X Z F F W G K L E F Q M J U M B G
E U R A D I O P H A R M A C E U T I C A L
S X V V I S U A L I Z A T I O N E B H E H
```

2. List some common tests used for screening health conditions.

3. Identify the secondary effects of nonradioactive agents.

4. Detail interventions to be taken for a client receiving a radiopaque agent.

Chapter 73   Poisons and Antidotes

1. Toxicology is the study of _____, _____, _____, and _____.

2. Poison is any substance that in _____ amounts can cause _____ or_____.

3. Toxidromes are _____.

4. Ipecac syrup is the most commonly used _____; it tastes _____.

5. Apomorphine is a/an _____ that causes _____.

6. Gastric lavage is _____.

7. Activated charcoal is instilled or swallowed following _____ or _____ to act as _____.

8. SLUDGE refers to the symptoms of _____, which are _____,_____, _____, _____, _____, and_____.

9. Describe the nurse's role in the emergency care of a client with a drug poisoning/overdose.

10. Match the sign to the toxin.

    ____ Convulsions or muscle twitching   a. Iron

    ____ Abdominal colic   b. Phenytoin

    ____ Bitter almond breath odor   c. Aspirin

    ____ Ataxia   d. Botulism

    ____ Salivation   e. Cyanide

    ____ Coma and drowsiness   f. Mercury

Answer Key

Chapter 1: Orientation to Pharmacology

1. d, f, b, c, a, e, g
2. Refer students to appropriate drug monographs.
3. assessment; nursing diagnosis; planning; implementation; evaluation
4. Cryptoquote: Enjoy the study of pharmacology!

Chapter 2: Legal and Ethical Aspects of Medication Administration

1. b, e, d, c, a
2. T, F, T, T
3. The medication order must be valid; the physician and nurse must be licensed; the nurse must know the purpose, actions, effects, and major side and toxic effects of the drug.
4. Word search key:

```
J  L  F  L  M  I  N  V  E  S  T  I  G  A  T  I  O  N  A  L
N  E  K  D  D  J  Q  B  A  J  K  S  R  E  D  R  O  A  L  R
M  G  K  Y  A  F  P  F  T  N  R  M  I  R  M  I  E  R  C  W
Z  E  A  W  S  X  E  O  Y  U  K  K  I  I  T  S  U  C  K  I
B  N  T  P  Q  G  X  M  O  R  T  R  P  A  T  B  N  O  I  D
D  D  Q  P  U  I  A  Z  U  S  J  Q  L  A  G  B  F  T  Z  A
V  Q  M  A  C  W  C  H  T  I  C  S  N  S  Y  N  E  I  J  P
Y  Z  R  I  J  L  M  I  Q  N  I  D  T  U  X  K  C  C  K  E
E  D  T  V  U  B  G  I  D  G  A  M  G  F  M  B  I  S  M  U
S  Y  H  B  V  Q  X  T  E  R  B  P  G  T  R  X  M  Z  W  C
B  I  Z  I  O  A  K  L  D  X  H  S  Q  M  F  P  O  J  N  Y
F  L  T  I  P  R  E  S  C  R  I  P  T  I  O  N  Z  G  M  I
```

Chapter 3: Principles of Drug Action

Across:

1. route
2. plasma
3. area
4. lung
5. TI
6. capsule
7. response
8. acidic
9. kinetics
10. age
11. lipid
12. cell
13. excretion

Down:

1. drugs
2. topical
3. iatrogenic
4. genetics
5. molecule
6. IM
7. kidney
8. stomach
9. sites
10. SQ
11. ASA
12. sex
13. oil
14. action

Chapter 4: Assessment, Nursing Diagnosis, and Planning

1. A, I, D, E, D, E, A, P, I, I, A, E, I
2. a. Stat: Demerol 100 mg intramuscularly now.
   b. RO: Milk of Magnesia 30 ml by mouth hour of sleep.
   c. prn: Seconal 100 mg by mouth hour of sleep as needed.
   d. RO: Lanoxin 0.25 mg by mouth every day.
   e. RO: Dilantin 100 mg by mouth.
3. A, T, S
4. monitor client's physiologic status; perform specific activities to manage and minimize the severity of the situation; consult with physician to obtain orders for appropriate interventions

Chapter 5: Implementation and Evaluation

1. a, g, c, f, i, k, j, l
2. 1 tbsp = ½ oz = 4 drams = 15 ml
3. 1 glassful = 240 ml = 8 oz
4. 3 tsp = 180 gtt
5. 0.5 gm = 500 mg
6. 2000 ml = 2 L
7. 1/7 dram = gr ix
8. 100 mg = 0.1 gm
9. 1 mg = 1000 micrograms
10. 16 oz = 1 lb
11. 120 grains = ii drams
12. 164 kg = 360.8 lb
13. 64 gal = 256 L
14. 6 cm = 0.06 m
15. a. 0.62 ml
    b. 2 ml
    c. gr 1/150 = 0.4 mg = 0.66 ml
16. 42 gtt
17. 50 gtt
18. crushed
19. deterioration
20. locked box or compartment; accounted for

Chapter 6: Cultural and Psychologic Aspects of Drug Therapy

1. b+d; c; d; e; b+d; a, a, b+d, a, b+d.
2. acupuncture, moxibustion, herbal remedies

3. Word search key:

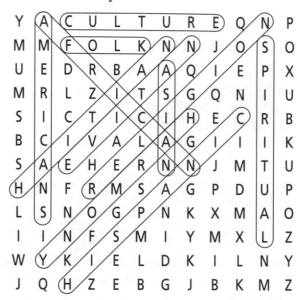

Chapter 7: Maternal and Child Drug Therapy

1. Gently massage area immediately anterior to the ear to facilitate entry of drops into ear canal. Before initial administration, assess whether child has excessive cerumen. If so, consult physician about its removal before instilling eardrops.
2.

Adult dose	Clark	BSA
atropine sulfate gr 1/150	gr 1/5	gr 1/5
aminophylline 0.5 gm	0.126 gm	0.2 gm
gentamycin 80 mg	15 mg	27 mg

3. a. Placenta
   b. Balance and advocate
4. a, e, b, d, c, a, c

Chapter 8: Drug Therapy for Older Adults

1. absorption (gastric pH; intestinal blood flow); distribution (lean body mass, adipose stores, total body water, serum albumin); metabolism (liver size, blood flow, functions); excretion (kidney function)
2. The elderly are living longer, have one or more chronic diseases, receive prescriptions from two or more prescribers, undergo physiologic changes, have limited income, on average use prescription and OTC drugs much more than general population, and are affected by polypharmacy.
3. This can be accomplished by a thorough assessment of the client's health status, current medica-

tion regimen, environmental factors, and implementation of appropriate interventions, client education, and counseling.

4. Review all medications with the client or caregiver; have the client or caregiver repeat the name, use, and dosing instructions for each; perform a func-

tions assessment to determine if client needs a compliance aid; discuss possible changes (simplification) with the prescriber if the drug regimen is complicated.

5. Scramble word grid answers:

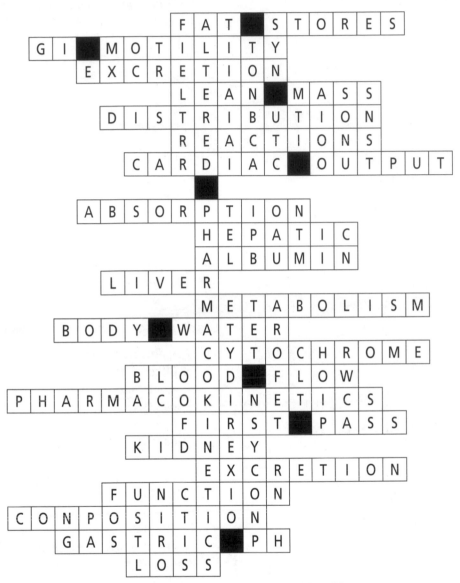

ANSWER: ALTERED PHARMACOKINETICS

Chapter 9: Substance Misuse and Abuse

Across:

1. psychic dependence
2. DAWN
3. misuse
4. hashish
5. ataxia
6. pills
7. coma
8. beer
9. cocaine
10. PCP
11. live
12. Nyquil
13. miosis

Down:

1. speedball
2. CNS
3. death
4. cough
5. anabolic
6. acne
7. brandy
8. LSD
9. priapism
10. abuse
11. flash
12. elation

Chapter 10: Client Education for Self-Administration of Medication

1. Word search key:

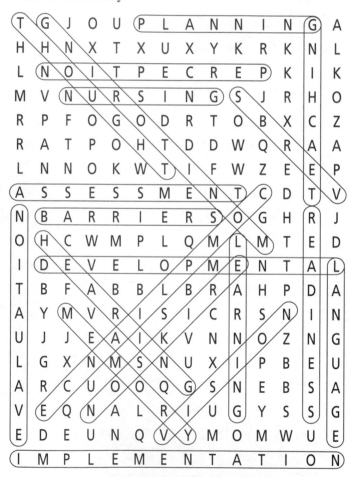

2. Answers should include some of the following: The client is chronically ill or on prolonged therapy. The client is relatively asymptomatic or feels better. Medication is expensive or inconvenient to obtain. Instructions are complex and not easily understood. Medication is unwieldy to take or has complicated mixing or measuring directions. Medicine tastes unpleasant or must be taken at inconvenient times or too many times a day. Plan contains many different medications, making drug-taking schedule complicated. Client has to wait longer than an hour in physician's office (correlated with noncompliance). Client does not understand or accept illness or its explanation; treatment plan does not fit client's concepts of health care. Client and care provider perceive clients' problems/goals in divergent ways. Client sees medication as contaminant or crutch on which dependence should be limited. Side effects are severe or inconvenient. Client has memory or visual impairment.

3. Goals should include "measurable" verbs such as *describe, discuss, list, relate, state, administer, demonstrate, perform, has an increase in,* etc. Students should avoid nonmeasurable verbs such as *accept, feel, appreciate, know,* and *understand.*

4. b, e, d, a, c, f

Chapter 11: Over-the-Counter Medications

1. a. A drug that relieves pain.
   b. Difficult fecal evacuation as a result of hard stools and perhaps infrequent bowel movements.
   c. A nursing diagnosis, the state in which an individual makes a self-diagnoses of constipation and ensures a daily bowel movement through the use of laxatives, enemas, and suppositories.

2. Refers to nomographs listing OTC drugs "generally recognized as safe and effective."

3. Do not give to children under age 17 without prescriber approval. Stop aspirin 5 to 7 days before surgery. Never put aspirin products directly on a tooth or gum surface. Do not take aspirin if it has a strong vinegar-like odor, which indicates deterioration. If stomach distress occurs, take aspirin with meals or food.

4. c, d, e, a, b, a, b, b, c, b

5. Adsorbents act by coating the walls of the GI tract, absorbing bacteria or toxins causing the diarrhea and expelling them with the stools.

6. CNS stimulation, insomnia, restlessness, dizziness, headaches, increased irritability

96

Chapter 12: Complementary and Alternative Pharmacology

1. i, e, b, k, a, d, j, f, c, h
2. Teaching should include that Lobelia does have agonist activities at nicotine receptors peripherally and centrally but that it is very toxic and can result in severe vomiting, pain, sweating, MI, and cardiovascular collapse leading to coma and death.
3. Cryptoquote: Homeopathy is a system of therapeutics.

Chapter 13: Overview of the Central Nervous System

1. nerve cells; astrocytes; brain's capillary walls
2. somatic motor pathway located in the CNS that affects skeletal muscles; coordination of muscle group movements and posture
3. consciousness and arousal effect; alerting mechanism; filter process that allows for concentration
4. acetylcholine
5. pain
6. cerebral stimulation
7. cerebrum
8. thalamus
9. mind; body
10. brainstem
11. glial cells; neurons
12. Dopamine, norepinephrine, and epinephrine. An increase in catecholamines causes cerebral stimulation. (Drugs that release catecholamines and reduce amine concentration in the brain have a depressing or sedative action.)
13. See Fig. 13-4, p. 251, in the text.

Chapter 14: Analgesics

1. Answers should include some of the following: seizures, tinnitus, jaundice (hepatic toxicity), pruritus, skin rash or facial edema (allergic reaction), breathing difficulties, respiratory depression, excitability (paradoxical reaction seen mainly in children), confusion, tachycardia
2. Gastric lavage or emesis; exchange transfusion, hemodialysis, peritoneal dialysis, or hemoperfusion may be necessary in severe overdose.
3. For mild pain (levels 1 to 3) administer a nonopioid and nonpharmacologic adjuvants; for moderate pain (levels 4 to 6) add a weak opioid combination with previous intervention; for severe pain (levels 7 to 10) administer strong opioids with nonpharmacologic adjuvants.

4. See Fig. 14-8, p. 269, in the text.

Chapter 15: Anesthetics

1. regional; local
2. a lower reported incidence of postoperative nausea, vomiting, and pain
3. inhaled; fat-soluble
4. analgesia; amnesia; muscular relaxation
5. a, a, b, c, b, b, c, d
6. Nursing plan should follow the general stages for an anesthetic but should include attention to the geriatric client's greater potential for drug interactions and side effects, an increased and prolonged drug effect, and mortality rates 4 to 8 times higher than normal.

Chapter 16: Antianxiety, Sedative, and Hypnotic Drugs

1. reduce feelings of anxiety
2. CNS depressant; CNS depression
3. paradoxical; dreaming
4. the elderly
5. The nurse should find out what a client's sleep habits are and how he or she ensures good sleep at home. A thorough sleep history is required including environmental control, physical self-care/relaxation, eating habits, and quiet recreation.
6. In addition to standard aspects of the nursing care plan for antianxiety drugs, the pediatric considerations should include references to the higher susceptibility of children to the CNS-depressant effects of benzodiazepines; danger of impaired functions with chronic use of clonazepam; the contraindications in children for buspirone, methyprylon, and, for hyperactive or psychotic children, diazepam; the importance of following manufacturer's dosage instructions; avoiding, when possible, concurrent use of other CNS depressants; monitoring excessive sedation, lethargy, or lack of coordination; monitoring for paradoxical reactions with use of barbiturates.
7. Interventions may include supportive nursing measures such as relaxation therapy, a back rub, reduction of environmental stimuli, or a warm drink.

Chapter 17: Anticonvulsants

1. Marked changes in the electrical activity of the cerebral cortex

2. apnea, respiratory depression, bronchospasms
3. all types of epilepsy except absence seizures
4. F, F, F
5. In addition to aspects of a general nursing care plan for anticonvulsants, pediatric considerations should include the following:

   Chewable phenytoin tablets are not indicated for once-daily administration.

   If skin rash develops with use of phenytoin, drug should be discontinued and physician should be notified.

   Intramuscular phenytoin injections should be avoided.

   If the mother received hydantoins during pregnancy, a neonate may require vitamin K to treat hypoprothrombinemia.

   There is increased susceptibility to gingival hyperplasia, especially with phenytoin or mephenytoin therapy.

   Coarse facial features and excessive body hair growth are more frequently reported in young clients.

   Impaired school performance is reported with high-dose, long-term hydantoin use.

   Whenever possible, other anticonvulsants should be considered before the hydantoins.

   Risk of serious hepatotoxicity exists with use of valproic acid or multiple anticonvulsant drug use
6. a, c, d, b

Chapter 18: Central Nervous System Stimulants

1. cerebral cortex
2. distractibility; short attention span; impulsive behavior; hyperactivity
3. daytime drowsiness; excessive sleep patterns
4. muscle weakness; narcolepsy
5. vivid auditory or visual dreams occurring at onset of sleep
6. The client should be instructed not to self-regulate the dose; habit-forming potential should be stressed. If effect seems to decrease, client should consult the prescriber. Instruct client to swallow sustained-release tablet without breaking, chewing, or crushing. Inform client of CNS and cardiovascular side effects; amphetamines may impair functioning in tasks requiring mental alertness and coordination. Caution client to store drug securely to avoid unintended use by another person.
7. More frequent: anorexia, increased nervousness, insomnia (usually more frequent in children). Less frequent: headache, nausea, abdominal pain, drowsiness, dizziness.

8. *CNS:* Increases alertness and decreases motor reaction time. Larger dosages may result in slowing of heart rate, vasoconstriction, and increased respiratory rate.

   Analgesic adjunct, vascular effect: Decreases cerebral blood flow and oxygen tension in the brain.

   Cardiovascular: Increases heart rate and cardiac output. Slightly slows or increases heart rate; overstimulation may cause tachycardia and cardiac irregularities. Appears to dilate peripheral blood vessels, thereby decreasing peripheral vascular resistance.

   Skeletal muscle: Increases contractual force and decreases muscle fatigue.

   Renal: Produces a mild diuretic effect.

   Gastrointestinal: Increases secretion of pepsin and hydrochloric acid from parietal cells.

   Respiratory: Appears to stimulate the medullary respiratory center.

   Additional effects: Increases metabolic activity; inhibits uterine contractions; increases glucose levels by stimulating glycolysis; and increases catecholamine levels in plasma and urine.

Chapter 19: Psychotherapeutic Drugs

1. c, a, d, b, b, a
2. See Box 19-2, Box 19-3, and Table 19-3.
3. See Box 19-6.
4. a. pseudoparkinsonism; b. akathisia; c. dystonia; d. tardive dyskinesia

Chapter 20: Overview of the Autonomic Nervous System

1. reflex arc
2. cholinergic neurons; cholinergic transmission
3. feedback control mechanism
4. smooth muscle, cardiac muscle, and glands of parasympathetic fibers and effector organs of the cholinergic sympathetic fibers
5. ganglia of both parasympathetic and sympathetic fibers, the adrenal medulla, and the skeletal (striated) muscle that is supplied by the somatic motor system
6. The parasympathetic system functions mainly to conserve energy and restore body resources of the organism, otherwise known as the system of rest and digestion. The sympathetic system mobilizes the organism during emergency and stress situations, so it is called the "fight or flight" system.
7. f, e, b, c, a, d

Chapter 21: Drugs Affecting the Parasympathetic Nervous System

1. sympathetic nervous system
2. parasympathetic nervous system
3. muscarinic effects of acetylcholine; anticholinergic
4. plant sources; synthesized; direct acting; indirect acting
5. acetylcholine; postganglionic; muscarine. Refer to Table 20-1 for complete list of muscarinic actions at various sites.
6. Acts by occupying the muscarinic (M) receptor sites, thereby preventing or reducing muscarinic response of acetylcholine. The drug-receptor complex is formed at the neuroeffector junctions of smooth muscle, cardiac muscle, and exocrine glands.
7. Atropine is indicated for the treatment of irritable bowel syndrome, spastic biliary tract disorders, and genitourinary disorders and as an antidote for cholinergic toxicity from excessive amounts of cholinesterase inhibitors, muscarinics, or organophosphate pesticide poisoning. It is also used to treat sinus bradycardia and Parkinson's disease, to prevent excessive salivation and respiratory tract secretions (preanesthetic), as an adjunctive medication for peptic ulcers, and for gastrointestinal radiography.
8. The client is instructed to slowly chew one piece of gum for about 30 minutes when the urge to smoke occurs. No more than 30 pieces are to be chewed in a day; the number chewed should be reduced each day over a 2- to 3-month period. Use for more than 3 months is not advised. At 6 months a gradual withdrawal program should be instituted.
   Nicotine gum may cause damage to dentures, inlays, fillings, and teeth. Client should use sugarless hard candies between doses of gum for oral stimulation and to relieve discomfort. If gum sticks to dental work, discontinue use and consult physician or dentist. Client should not smoke while being treated. Nicotine gum must be used under medical supervision, combined with a supervised program for smoking cessation.
9. Remove patch from sealed pouch just before application. Remove protective liner from sticky side of patch, and touching this side as little as possible, apply patch to selected skin site. Press patch to skin with palm for about 10 seconds. Fold previously used patch in half with sticky side together and place in newly opened pouch of replacement patch. Throw pouch away. Wash hands immediately.
10. Client is at risk for hyperthermia related to suppression of sweat gland activity; potential for injury related to allergic reaction, blurred vision, dizziness, or lightheadedness; altered thought processes (confusion); altered comfort related to dry mouth or increased sensitivity of eyes to light; urinary retention related to the drug's anticholinergic effects; altered bowel elimination pattern (constipation) related to decreased motility of the GI tract.

Chapter 22: Drugs Affecting the Sympathetic (Adrenergic) Nervous System

1. a, c — a, d, d, a, c, a, b
2. More frequent: systemic reactions such as increased nervousness, restlessness; insomnia. Less frequent: elevation of blood pressure, tachycardia, tremors, sweating, nausea, vomiting, pallor, weakness. Inhalation reactions: bronchial irritation and coughing (usually with high doses), dry mouth and throat, headaches, red or flushing face or skin.
3. inotropic; chronotropic; dromotropic
4. noncompetitive, long-acting antagonists; competitive, short-acting antagonists; ergot alkaloids
5. Refer to drug monograph for complete listing of possible answers.

Chapter 23: Drugs for Specific CNS-Peripheral Dysfunctions

1. A progressively debilitating disorder of the CNS caused by a degeneration of the dopamine-producing neurons of the substantia nigra, which produces a dopamine/acetylcholine imbalance. Symptoms include muscle rigidity and muscle tremor. The muscle rigidity or increased tone appears as "ratchet resistance" or "cogwheel rigidity." The muscle tremors appear to have a "to-and-fro" movement and are usually worse at rest and commonly manifested as "pill-rolling" motion of the hands and bobbing of the head.
2. These drugs, which inhibit or block the effects of acetylcholine, are referred to as anticholinergic drugs. They block central cholinergic excitatory pathways, returning the dopamine/acetylcholine balance in the brain (especially in the basal ganglia) to normal.
3. Administer before meals. For geriatric clients and individuals receiving other medications, the dosage of levodopa should be titrated to reach the client's therapeutic levels with minimum side effects.

4. A progressive and presently incurable disease characterized by the loss of, or decrease in, acetylcholine receptors caused by an autoimmune process resulting in skeletal muscle weakness and fatigue. The most common early reported symptoms are ptosis and diplopia. Dysarthria, dysphagia, and limb weakness, especially of the upper extremities, also occur in advanced stages. Client may complain of shoulder fatigue after shaving or combing hair or of hand weakness.

5. Answers should include two of the following:
   Guanadrel, guanethidine, mecamylamine, trimethaphan: May antagonize action of cholinesterase inhibitor drugs, resulting in increased muscle weakness, respiratory muscle weakness, and difficulty swallowing.
   Procainamide: May antagonize action of cholinesterase inhibitor drugs.
   Other cholinesterase inhibitors: Serious additive toxicity may result.

6. With short-term (1 to 3 days' use) or chronic oral intake of dantrolene: mild diarrhea, dizziness, sleepiness, feelings of uncomfortableness or unusual fatigue, muscle weakness (not of respiratory muscles), nausea, or vomiting.

7. In addition to the nursing management discussed as appropriate to centrally acting skeletal muscle relaxant therapy in general, baclofen requires the following considerations:
   Dosage should be increased gradually.

A gradual reduction in dosage over a period of 2 weeks is recommended.

Tell the client that maximum benefit may not be reached for 1 to 2 months.

Alert the client to possible side effects. If orthostatic hypotension is a concern, instruct the client to come to an upright position slowly.

Administration of baclofen may increase the client's blood glucose levels, requiring an adjustment of insulin dosage during therapy and when baclofen therapy is stopped.

Geriatric clients are at risk for adverse CNS reactions.

Epileptic clients are at risk for increased seizure activity.

Monitor the client's clinical state and EEG results during therapy.

Chapter 24: Overview of the Cardiovascular System

Across:

1. vagal	5. two	10. heart
2. ATP	6. Ca	11. calcium
3. Frank-Starling	7. velocity	12. threshold
4. Purkinje	8. block	13. ions
	9. systole	

Down:

1. Na	4. repolarization	8. EKG
2. atria	5. acetylcholine	9. QRS
3. ventricles	6. glycosides	10. His
	7. AV	

1. Word search key:

```
G N C P S F L K O A M R T S Q D W V K X
Y L S E R Z Z L Q W H F O Z X Z H V I K
O S R W E J G K P J A B X W C L B Q L R
O U W V K Y X U A C V L I E R H P E S R
M B P X A H A Y H S Q Z C K R N R Z I U
R Y F O M C X K K C F Z I G J B J Y Z V
J I F E E W J W R M J A T L X Z W Z W V
F H A O C E D X H B G L Y C O S I D E B
G E M Y A H W A L V E C R H D L B M I Y
H N R G P W F Z G Q N P I R J E X C E K
N O I T A L L I R B I F O O Z V C M N O
U N N S O A F D G Z X M U N I X O G I D
R I O U R U V P I N O T R O P I C Y H J
K R N V R U U J M T N A P T X R T D Y Z
T L E S P N N F R D A J E R Y E K T J Q
Q I J J K E X O C O L M B O A I B J Y O
X M Q W U D P Y O N G F A P Z N R O C Q
G M N R R I D I G I T A L I Z A T I O N
W O B R C B D P V Q Q B W C O Z X B Q K
J W W W J B H Y J U Y W J B Y X J Z X W
```

2. Answers should include three of the following: potassium loss (through hypokalemia, poor dietary intake, adrenal steroid use, or surgical procedures associated with severe electrolyte disturbances); hypercalcemia; pathologic conditions such as kidney, liver, and severe heart disease.

3. Incomplete AV block, increasing age; clients with electronic pacemakers; electrolyte imbalances; ventricular dysrhythmias; myocardial pathology; conduction disorders; myxedema, severe pulmonary disease, or carotid sinus hypersensitivity

4. Instruct client to take digitalis at the same time each day, precisely as prescribed. Do not skip or double a dose if missed. Do not change brand. Inform client that digoxin and Lanoxin are essentially the same drug. If using elixir form, dose should be determined using special dropper. Caution client not to take other medications without prior approval of physician.

Restrict sodium intake to 2 g daily. Report weight gain of 1 or 2 pounds a day; avoid licorice.

Advise client to carry medical identification and to alert health professionals unfamiliar with drug regimen that the drug is being taken.

Teach client how to take pulse before each dose. Dose should be withheld and physician notified if the pulse is below 60 or above 110 and/or is erratic or if client suffers from anorexia, diarrhea, nausea, vomiting, sudden weight gain, or apparent edema. Visual disturbances should be reported.

5. Altered comfort, nausea, vomiting, abdominal pain; hyperpyrexia; potential complications of decreased cardiac output, dysrhythmias, dose-dependent thrombocytopenia, hepatotoxicity, and hypersensitivity reactions

Chapter 26: Antidysrhythmics

1. Cryptoquote: Dysrhythmia is caused by a disorder affecting the cells of the conduction system or myocardium.
2. a, b, g, a, e, c, f, b, f, d
3. F, T, F, T

Chapter 27: Antihypertensives

1. Mechanism that regulates blood pressure by increasing or decreasing blood volume through kidney function. When blood flow through the kidneys is reduced, reduced renal arterial pressure causes release of renin into the circulation. Renin catalyzes cleavage of a plasma protein to form angiotensin I, which is converted by angiotensin-converting enzyme (ACE) to angiotensin II.
   Angiotensin II stimulates secretion of aldosterone, which promotes reabsorption of sodium by kidneys. The increased sodium elevates osmotic pressure in the plasma and a release of antidiuretic hormone from the hypothalamus. Angiotensin II acts on the kidney tubules to promote reabsorption of water.
   Excessive fluid retention is controlled by negative-feedback mechanism operating within this system so that fluid balance is restored to a normal level. Thus the renin-angiotensin-aldosterone system involves slow adjustments to changes in fluid volume.
2. diuretics, calcium antagonists
3. Older adults have increased risk of CV morbidity and mortality. Nonpharmacologic means of blood pressure reduction are indicated.
   Antihypertensive drugs should be started with smaller than usual doses, increased by smaller than usual amounts, and scheduled at less frequent intervals, since the elderly are more sensitive to volume depletion and sympathetic inhibition than younger clients. They commonly have impaired CV reflexes, making them more susceptible to hypotension.
   In clients with isolated systolic hypertension who are treated with antihypertensive drugs, the systolic pressure should be cautiously decreased to 140 to 160 mm Hg. Only if this medication level is tolerated without side effects should consideration be given to further lowering the systolic value. The elderly client's response to both nonpharmacologic and pharmacologic therapies should be monitored closely.
4. T, T, T, F

5. *Routes:* oral, transdermal
   Distribution: wide throughout body, passes blood-brain barrier
   Dosage: initial dose 0.1 mg bid, then increased by 0.1 to 0.2 mg every 2-4 days until B/P under control
   Action: stimulates central alpha 2 receptors
   Adverse effects: dry mouth, headaches, constipation, weakness, postural hypotension, impotency or decreased sexual drive, insomnia, anxiety, anorexia, nausea, vomiting, pruritus
   Nursing diagnoses: risk for injury; impaired skin integrity; fluid volume excess related to sodium and water retention; sleep pattern disturbance; constipation; altered oral mucous membranes; fatigue; sexual dysfunction; altered comfort; altered thought processes. See Nursing Care Plan for more.

Chapter 28: Calcium Channel Blockers

1. an action potential without an external stimulus
2. antianginal; antidysrhythmic; antihypertensive
3. peripheral vascular resistance; blood pressure
4. Answers should include two of the following:
   Beta-adrenergic blockers: bradycardia, hypotension, and heart failure caused by prolonged AV conduction
   Carbamazepine: increased serum levels
   Cyclosporine: increased serum levels (to toxic levels)
   Digitalis glycosides: increased serum levels
   Disopyramide: additive negative inotropic effects, sometimes fatal
5. More frequent: dizziness, headaches, nausea, feelings of warmth or flushing. Less frequent: constipation.
6. Answers should include five of the following:
   Instruct client to perform meticulous daily dental hygiene.
   Instruct client to keep a record of nitroglycerin administration and anginal episodes and report promptly if changes occur.
   Instruct client to move from a sitting or lying position to a standing position cautiously.
   Advise client to avoid alcohol.
   Emphasize importance of regular visits to a health care provider.
   Teach client to take a pulse and report a heart rate of less than 50.
   Instruct client to report headaches, rashes, nausea, vomiting, edema, and weight gain.
   Advise client to take missed dose as soon as it is remembered, unless it is time for next dose.

If drugs are being taken as antihypertensives, instruct client to take medication even if feeling well. Advise client regarding hazards of untreated hypertension and need for decreased sodium intake, smoking cessation, and weight control.

Caution client to check with prescriber before taking other medications.

For verapamil injection, instruct client to remain recumbent following IV bolus for at least 1 hour.

7. Use IV atropine, isoproterenol, norepinephrine, or calcium chloride. An electronic cardiac pacemaker may be necessary.

Chapter 29: Vasodilators and Antihemorrheologic Agents

1. pain below the sternum; exercise or stress; rest
2. their effect on the veins and arteries
3. carbon monoxide hemoglobin; available blood oxygen
4. an insufficient blood supply to skeletal muscles in the legs; Buerger's disease
5. F, T, F
6. Instruct client to place the tablet between upper lip and gum to dissolve and above incisors if food or drink is to be taken within 3 to 5 hours. Caution against using at bedtime, since aspiration is a risk. The tablet may be replaced if it is accidentally swallowed.
7. To decrease duration and intensity of pain during an attack; to prophylactically decrease frequency of attacks and improve work capacity even though angina may occur; to prevent or delay the onset of myocardial infarction
8. It improves microcirculation of ischemic tissues by inhibiting phosphodiesterase, which increases cyclic AMP, and it lowers blood viscosity by decreasing fibrinogen concentration and inhibiting aggregation of RBCs and platelets.

Chapter 30: Overview of the Blood

Across:

1. leukocytes	5. HCT	9. thrombocytes
2. albumin	6. factor	10. RH
3. hemoglobin	7. fibrin	11. PLT
4. plasma	8. anemia	

Down:

1. erythropoietin	4. alpha	8. blood
2. stasis	5. neutrophils	9. clot
3. lymph	6. ABO	10. types
	7. oxygen	

Chapter 31: Anticoagulants, Thrombolytics, and Blood Components

1. b, b, a, a, a, b
2. a, b, b, a, a, b, a, b
3. apprehension, restlessness, fever, chills, head or back pain, rash, hypotension, nausea and vomiting, dyspnea, cyanosis
4. Increased risk of bleeding and hemorrhage. Heparin has been administered with thrombolytic agents to treat an acute coronary arterial occlusion.
5. Refer to box titled *Implications for the Older Adult: Anticoagulants.*

Chapter 32: Antihyperlipidemic Drugs

1. metabolic; increased concentrations of cholesterol and triglycerides
2. high levels of circulating triglycerides and cholesterol
3. cholesterol and triglycerides; the body cells of membranes; the liver
4. lipid compounds; plasma proteins; densities and electrophoretic mobilities
5. cholesterol; the most harmful
6. largest; dense; the small intestine during absorption of a fatty meal
7. Answers should include two of the following drugs and their effects:
   Oral anticoagulants, coumarins, indanediones: decrease absorption of oral anticoagulants and vitamin K.
   Digitalis glycosides, especially digitoxin: half-life of digitalis glycosides and GI absorption may be reduced.
   Thiazide diuretics (oral), oral propranolol, oral penicillin G, oral tetracyclines, oral vancomycin: decreased absorption of these medications has been reported.
   Thyroid hormones: decreased absorption of thyroid products is reported.
8. Before initiating clofibrate therapy, advise client to adhere to diet prescribed by physician. Encourage weight reduction and physical exercise.

Warn client that a paradoxical rise may occur in 2 or 3 months, but afterward a further decrease is customary.

Instruct client to keep clinical appointments. If serum cholesterol and triglyceride levels are not lowered within 3 months, drug therapy is usually discontinued.

Advise client to report flu-like symptoms. Instruct individual to check with physician about alcohol intake since its use may be restricted to prevent hypertriglyceridemia.

9. flatulence, stomach pain, nausea, diarrhea or constipation, headaches

Chapter 33: Overview of the Urinary System

1. See Figs. 33-1 and 33-4, pp. 664 and 666, in the textbook.
2. a, a, a, e, b, b, c, d, a
3. a. Hypertonic describes a solution that has more solids to a prescribed amount of fluid; usually 100 ml. The general rule of thumb is that the percent of a solution represents the amount of solids in grams to 100 ml of fluid. Example: Isotonic solution is 0.9% (900 mg of sodium chloride to 100 ml water), thus a hypertonic solution would be 3% saline/water (3 gm/100 ml).
   b. Hypotonic describes a solution that has fewer solids to a prescribed amount of fluid. Example: 0.45% normal saline.

Chapter 34: Diuretics

1. c, a, b, b, a, c
2. commonly; hypertension; cirrhosis; nephrotic syndrome; congestive heart failure; electrolyte; tubular; kidney
3. c — d — a — d — c, d — b, d — a, b — a — d
4. Refer to box titled *Geriatric Implications: Diuretics* for complete coverage of considerations.

Chapter 35: Uricosuric Drugs

1. metabolic; acute pain; swelling; tenderness
2. hyperuricemia; uric acid in the blood
3. deposits of uric acid or urates which form in cartilage
4. enzyme necessary to convert hypoxanthine to xanthine and xanthine to uric acid
5. To end the acute gouty attack as soon as possible; to prevent recurrence of acute gouty arthritis; to prevent formation of uric acid stones in the kidneys;

to reduce or prevent disease complications that result from sodium urate deposits in joints and kidneys
6. Inhibits secretion of weak organic acids at both the proximal and the distal renal tubules in the kidneys
7. T, T, T, T, F
8. You should have designed a sheet or card, using the drug interactions in the probenecid monograph, rewording and simplifying the information in layperson's terms.

Chapter 36: Drug Therapy for Renal System Dysfunction

1. decline; 5
2. irreversible
3. urea in the blood
4. hemodialysis; peritoneal dialysis; organ transplantation
5. electrolytes; wastes; osmosis; diffusion; filtration
6. Serum creatinine and blood urea nitrogen (BUN) levels. The creatinine level, which is related to muscle mass, is independent of protein consumption and is a more accurate measure of renal function than is the BUN.
7. Most common: increasing weakness, fatigue, lethargy. GI signs: anorexia, GI distress, nausea, vomiting, thirst, weight loss. Paresthesias, peripheral neuropathy, convulsions, and neuromuscular irritability may also occur. On examination, the client may appear pale and dehydrated and have an increased respiratory rate and uremic breath. Hypertension with retinopathy, cardiac hypertrophy, pulmonary edema, or pericarditis may often be present.
8. Epoetin alfa is a glycoprotein chemically identical to human erythropoietin. It is indicated for treatment of anemia associated with renal failure and severe anemia associated with AIDS.
   Epoetin alfa has the same biologic action as the endogenous hormone; it stimulates erythropoiesis in the bone marrow and also induces the release of reticulocytes from bone marrow. Since endogenous erythropoietin is manufactured mainly in the kidneys, anemia resulting from chronic renal failure is caused by inadequate production of the hormone.
9. Drug dosage may be decreased (dosage reduction method) while maintaining the usual interval, or if the dosage is the usually prescribed dose, the interval between doses is lengthened (interval extension method). Usually the dosage reduction method is preferred for drugs that require a constant blood therapeutic level.

10. Refer to Table 36-1 for complete list of possible answers.
11. Word search key:

```
A C K S D A X E D Q Q Q R Y Y
S N O I T N E V R E T N I A E
T N W S D T E X Q F H G H H A
O G S Y A N Q J W K G K R P P
R X H L L A E N O T I R E P A
D Q L A N E R Y U K E W T L C
L G N I S R U N G K W B M N U
X R Z D A B K Q N L I F C T X
H Z X O E J R W Z T C I E E J
H N B M U A B F A I L U R E F
H B E E L U C H R O N I C L D
C D S H N M A U D E V D U H C
T R G A E A Z O T E M I A T R
B N X C M R S D P E D A W V E
F A K C P I S O B U B G M S A
O P N X N L E D Y P Y N X G T
Y X B G E T Y Q R D P O G Q I
G S Q V I H R O D U D S R Z N
V M C N D T T V N U G I O A I
V G F R A R E Z D C O S T U N
U X Q N O I T A U L A V E S E
```

Chapter 37: Overview of the Respiratory System

1. Alveolus key:

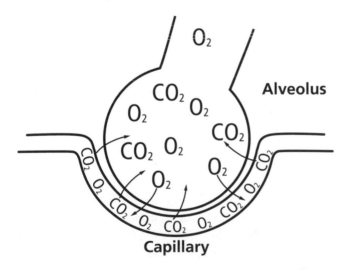

2. Shape and size of each portion of the respiratory tract; presence of ciliated, mucus-secreting, epithe-lial lining throughout most of the respiratory tract; character and thickness of respiratory tract secretions; compliance of the cartilaginous and bony supports; pressure gradients; traction on airway walls; absence of foreign substances in the lumen of the respiratory tract

3. The tracheobronchial tree is innervated by the autonomic nervous system. The bronchial smooth muscle tone is influenced by the balance maintained between parasympathetic and sympathetic stimuli during rest. Activation of the parasympathetic fiber (vagus nerve) releases acetylcholine, which results in bronchoconstriction and narrowing of the airway. By contrast, the stimulation of the sympathetic fiber and the sympathoadrenal system releases epinephrine and norepinephrine from the adrenal medulla into circulation. Their action on the beta$_2$ receptor sites in the bronchial smooth muscle produces bronchodilation by means of smooth muscle relaxation.

4. Basic rhythm for respiration is initiated and maintained in the medullary rhythmicity area located beneath the lower part of the floor of the fourth ventricle in the medial half of the medulla. Neurons that control inspiration and expiration intermingle and discharge, or fire impulses, alternately. However, signals from the spinal cord, the cerebral cortex and midbrain, the apneustic area of the pons, and the pneumotaxic area of the upper pons can enter the medullary rhythmicity area, modify the rhythm of respiration, and contribute to the normal pattern of respiration.

Chapter 38: Mucokinetic, Bronchodilator, and Antiasthmatic Drugs

1. abnormal or excessive respiratory tract secretions; sputum retention
2. phlegm; abnormal, or viscous; the lower respiratory tree; mucus
3. inhaled, or topical; pulmonary nebulization
4. expectorants; destructive
5. chronic pulmonary diseases
6. Relax smooth muscle, particularly bronchial muscle; stimulate cardiac muscle and the CNS; produce diuresis
7. Bronchodilation and pulmonary decongestion; loosening of secretions; topical applications of steroids; moistening, cooling, or heating of inspired air
8. Start within 10 to 12 hours after ingestion of overdose for most benefit, but it is still beneficial if started within the first 24 hours. Support client

through gastric lavage, induced emesis, or other appropriate therapies. Monitor liver function studies and plasma acetaminophen concentrations for potential hepatotoxicity. Monitor the client with knowledge deficit or a high risk for self-harm.

9. Traditionally asthma was classified on the basis of stimuli that may induce an attack. However, since many asthmatic individuals have a combination of causative factors, this type of classification is not considered useful. Instead clients are now classified according to frequency and severity.

10. Most frequent: nervousness, insomnia, tachycardia. Less frequent: dizziness, headaches, hypotension, anorexia, nausea, pounding tachycardia, sweating, vomiting, dry mouth and throat, difficulty in urination. Rare adverse reactions: breathing difficulties, chest pain.

11. (1) Fully insert canister into shell, remove cap, and shake.

(2) Exhale fully.

(3) Place mouthpiece over the tongue in the mouth. Close lips tightly and press top of canister firmly, simultaneously inhaling deeply through the mouth (with some models, mouthpiece should be held 1 or 2 inches from open mouth).

(4) Hold breath and inhale as long as possible.

(5) Release pressure, remove inhaler, and breathe slowly. Wait 1 full minute before administering second puff. Repeat steps.

12. T, T, F

13. Keep house as dust free as possible and avoid shag carpeting, heavy draperies, dust on silk flower arrangements, use of perfumed soap and products, and smokers or smoke-contaminated areas

Chapter 39: Oxygen and Miscellaneous Respiratory Agents

1. arterial blood oxygen saturation
2. hypoxemia
3. hypoxia; brain
4. COPD; hypercapnia
5. increased respiratory rate; oxygen therapy
6. colorless; odorless; tasteless; life
7. colorless; odorless; respiration; circulation; the CNS
8. Nasal catheter; nasal cannula; oxygen mask; simple face mask; partial rebreathing mask; nonrebreathing mask; Ventimask
9. Advise client to: maintain dental hygiene and checkups; ease dry mouth with ice, sugarless gum, or hard candy; use caution driving or operating hazardous equipment; report symptoms of blood dyscrasias; avoid ingestion of alcohol or CNS depressants. As prophylaxis for motion sickness, the drug must be taken 30 minutes to 1 or 2 hours before effect is needed. These drugs interfere with allergy skin tests.

10. T, F, F, F, T

Chapter 40: Overview of the Gastrointestinal Tract

1. mechanical; chemical; digestion
2. swallowing
3. dysphagia
4. food bolus; GI tract; band contraction
5. inflammation of the gallbladder; gallstones
6. mouth; anus
7. a, c, b, f, d, h, e, c, e, g, d, e
8. External innervation of the GI system is supplied by the divisions of the autonomic nervous system, which correlate activities between different regions of the GI system and also between this system and other parts of the body.

Chapter 41: Drugs Affecting the Gastrointestinal Tract

1. A, B, A, H, N, H
2. Store out of reach in a safe area, preferably a locked cabinet. Use of mouthwash is not recommended since children often swallow the mouthwash rather than expectorate it.
3. c+b, d, a, a, b
4. Administer oral form 30 minutes before meals and at bedtime; administer IV injections slowly over 1 to 2 minutes; infusions should not be for a period of less than 15 minutes. Keep solutions of parenteral dosage for 48 hours after dilution; protect from light; discard unused portions after 48 hours. Do not give in combination with drugs having extrapyramidal side effects. Extrapyramidal side effects may be seen at therapeutic doses and are more likely to occur in children and young adults.
5. Diarrhea, headache
6. *H. pylori* is a bacteria that increases a client's chance for gastritis and gastric and duodenal ulcers.
7. See *Geriatric Implications* within the text.
8. They inhibit the hydrogen/potassium ATPase enzyme system at the secretory surface of the gastric parietal cells, thus suppressing gastric acid secretion.
9. Altered bowel elimination (diarrhea); altered comfort.

10. Increased fluids, vegetables, fruits, and bran products. Malt soup extract is often suggested for infants up to 2 months old.
11. Refer to the Nursing Care Plan in your textbook, p. 782.

Chapter 42: Overview of the Eye

1. receptor; vision
2. anterior; transparent; light
3. constriction; miosis
4. dilation; mydriasis
5. changes shape; in sharp focus
6. transparency; opaque; cataract
7. Paralysis of the ciliary muscle
8. Interfere with cholinesterase activity; act like acetylcholine at receptor sites in the sphincter muscle
9. Interfere with action of acetylcholine; stimulate sympathetic or adrenergic receptors
10. Bathes and feeds the lens, iris, and posterior surface of the cornea
11. Ciliary muscle contraction; ability of the lens to assume a more biconvex shape when tension on the ligaments is relaxed
12. Rods, cones
13. Eyelashes, eyelids, blinking, tears

Chapter 43: Ophthalmic Drugs

1. abnormally elevated intraocular pressure (IOP); irreversible blindness
2. glaucoma; accommodative esotropia (crossed eyes)
3. enzymatic destruction of acetylcholine; inactivating cholinesterase
4. *Conjunctivitis:* acute inflammation of the conjunctiva
   Hordeolum: acute localized infection of the eyelash follicles and glands of the anterior lid margin
   Chalazion: infection of the meibomian (sebaceous) glands of the eyelids
   Keratitis: corneal inflammation caused by bacterial infection
   Uveitis: infection of the uveal tract, or vascular layer of the eye
5. Primary, secondary, congenital
6. Knowledge deficit related to new ophthalmic drug regimen; anxiety related to possible decrease in or loss of vision; alteration in comfort related to ophthalmic disorder; potential injury related to impaired vision
7. Refer to Table 43-2 for complete listing.
8. Refer to box titled *Guidelines for Instillation of Eyedrops and Ointments.*
9. Bradycardia, syncope, low blood pressure, asthmatic attack, congestive heart failure, hallucinations, loss of appetite, headaches, nausea, weakness, depression

Chapter 44: Overview of the Ear

1. thin, transparent partition of tissue; canal; middle ear
2. middle ear; nasopharynx; the individual swallows, chews, yawns, or moves the jaw
3. malleus; incus; stapes; sound waves
4. cochlea
5. *External ear:* outer ear (pinna), external auditory canal
   Middle ear: auditory ossicles (malleus, incus, and stapes)
   Inner ear: bony labyrinth (vestibule, cochlea, semicircular canals), membranous labyrinth
6. Connects middle ear to nasopharynx. The eustachian tube equalizes air pressure on both sides of the eardrum to prevent the eardrum from rupturing.
7. otitis media
8. a, c, b, b, c

Chapter 45: Drugs Affecting the Ear

1. Burning, redness, rash, swelling, or other signs of topical irritation that were not present before the start of therapy
2. (1) Assess (a) hearing and symptoms, (b) that ear canal is clear and that tympanic membrane is intact, (c) for improper hygiene or practices.
   (2) Run warm water over bottle or immerse it in warm water.
   (3) Let an irritable child get comfortable. Cleanse any drainage and position affected ear upward.
   (4) In children 3 years or younger, gently pull pinna slightly down and back to instill drops. In older children and adults, hold pinna up and back. Gently massage area immediately anterior to the ear to facilitate entry.
   (5) Instruct client to remain on his or her side for 5 minutes, using a cotton pledget if desired. Alert client to the hazard of temporary impaired hearing related to therapy.
3. Serum levels of some drugs may be monitored. Monitor client's ability to hear by observing cues and noting client's comments on hearing ability. Report indications of increased hearing loss to the

prescriber. When given IV, aminoglycosides should be administered over 30 to 60 minutes to avoid high peak levels. Instruct clients to report tinnitus or any other hearing impairment immediately.

4. Refer to Table 45-1 in text for listing.
5. Refer to Table 45-2 in text for listing.

Chapter 46: Overview of the Endocrine System

1. See Fig. 46-1, p. 820, in the textbook.
2. Secretory and motor activities of the digestive tract; energy production; composition and volume of extracellular fluid; adaptation, such as acclimatization and immunity; growth and development; reproduction and lactation
3. a, e, d, a, a, b, f, e, e, c, a, f, b

Chapter 47: Drugs Affecting the Pituitary

1. Word search key:

2. Most frequent: pain at injection site (usually with tannate dosage form). Less frequent: stomach gas and pain, diarrhea, dizziness, increased pressure for bowel evacuation, nausea, vomiting, tremors, sweating, pallor.
3. Obtain baseline data from bone age determinations, thyroid function studies, and anti–growth hormone antibody; monitor periodically. Pain and swelling have occurred at the site of injection. After several months of therapy, antibodies to somatrem may be formed in some clients. These rarely reduce the response to therapy. Monitor for signs of hypothyroidism. Dilute for parenteral use with 1 to 5 ml diluent provided. Do not shake vial; rotate gently until clear. Do not use cloudy solution. Store in refrigerator. Advise client to visit endocrinologist regularly.
4. Hepatitis and AIDS as a result of shared needles and syringes

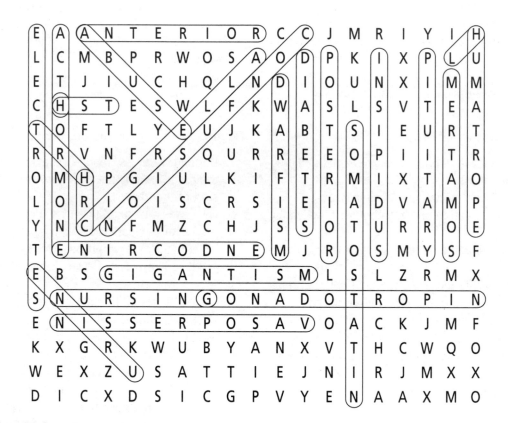

Chapter 48: Drugs Affecting the Parathyroid and Thyroid

1. primary hyperparathyroidism
2. thyroid replacement therapy
3. antithyroid; thyroid release from hyperfunctioning thyroid gland
4. hypothyroidism
5. radioactive iodine; clients who are poor surgical risks, those with advanced cardiac disease, and elderly clients
6. a, c, b, a, a, d, b, b, b, c, a
7. Vitamin D and calcium supplements. Calcitriol is an active metabolite form of vitamin D.
8. Protirelin and thyrotropin
9. Instruct client in appropriate methods for disposal of urine and feces. If client is discharged but radiation precautions are still necessary, ensure that the client receives specific instruction. If the client received dosage of ^{131}I for hyperthyroidism or thyroid carcinoma, these 48- to 72-hour precautions may include the following: avoiding close contact with others, especially children; not kissing anyone or sharing others' eating or drinking utensils; washing sink and tub after use; using and washing clothes, towels, and linens separately.

Chapter 49: Drugs Affecting the Adrenal Cortex

1. hormones; glucocorticoids; mineralocorticoids
2. daily (24-hour); dark/light and sleep/wakefulness cycles
3. periodic or intermittent; once every 24 hours
4. corticosteroids; blood sugar; emergency actions
5. Answers should include any three of the following: antiinflammatory action; maintenance of normal blood pressure; carbohydrate and protein metabolism; fat metabolism; thymolytic, lympholytic, and eosinopenic actions; stress effects.
6. *GI:* abdominal pains, black tarry stools (GI bleeding)
   Immune: lowers resistance to infections; may also mask symptoms of infections
   Musculoskeletal: hip or shoulder pain; muscle cramping or pain; increased weakness; muscle weakness; bone pain
7. See chart in Assessment section under *Nursing Management: Mineralocorticoid Therapy.*
8. Use antiadrenals cautiously in clients undergoing stress such as surgery, infection, trauma, and acute illness. Do not administer to clients with recent exposure to chickenpox and herpes zoster. Do not give to pregnant women. Geriatric clients may be more sensitive to the drug's CNS effects. Obtain baseline lying and standing blood pressures, serum electrolyte levels, thyroid function studies, and AST (SGOT) concentrations.

Chapter 50: Drugs Affecting the Pancreas

1. insulin; glucagon
2. glycogenolysis; gluconeogenesis
3. Mark first injection site with spot bandage and give future injections around bandage. Imagine circle as a clock, administering injections at 12, 3, 6, and 9 o'clock points before starting new circle more than an inch away from previous sites. Administer 5 injections per circle.
4. Answers should include five of the following: 3 glucose tablets, 4 oz orange juice, 6 oz regular soda, 6-8 oz 2% fat or skim milk, 6-8 Life-Savers, 3 graham cracker squares, 6 jelly beans, 2 tablespoons raisins, 1 small (2 oz) tube of cake frosting
5. They enhance the release of insulin from beta cells in the pancreas, decrease liver glycogenolysis and gluconeogenesis, and increase the sensitivity to insulin in body tissues. Therefore they reduce blood glucose concentration in persons with a functioning pancreas.
6. Protect vials from heat and cold; store in cool place, but do not freeze. Do not store U-500 insulin with other insulin preparations. Vials of insoluble preparations should be rotated between the hands and inverted end-to-end several times before a dose is withdrawn. A vial should not be shaken vigorously or the suspension made to foam. Do not interchange human, beef, or pork insulins. Use properly calibrated syringe for insulin; avoid bubbles.
   Administer subcutaneously with 25- or 26-gauge needle. Administer at 90-degree angle in large fold of pinched skin or insert at 30- to 45-degree angle at base of fold of skin. Apply pressure but do not rub. Rotate injection sites.
   Adsorption on tubing surface requires client monitoring of insulin needs. Saturation of adsorption sites on tubing requires special care. Minimize adsorption by injecting directly into vein, using intermittent infusion device, or using port close to IV access site. When insulin is administered as an infusion, use IV pump.
7. b, a, a, b, b, b, a
8. Glucagon is released to maintain plasma levels of glucose by stimulating hepatic glycogenolysis and gluconeogenesis and by inhibition of glycogen synthesis. Glucagon's effect is accelerated by stimula-

tion of synthesis of cyclic AMP (cAMP). Glucagon is indicated for the treatment of hypoglycemia in clients with diabetes and as an adjunct for gastrointestinal radiography. It is effective only if liver glycogen is available.

Chapter 51: Overview of the Female and Male Reproductive Systems

Across:

1. follicle
2. parasympathetic
3. LH
4. gonads
5. prostate
6. testosterone
7. sperm
8. orgasm
9. ejaculation
10. vasectomy

Down:

1. ova
2. ICSH
3. ovary
4. LTH
5. progesterone
6. estrogens
7. climacteric
8. semen
9. uterus
10. labia
11. penis

Chapter 52: Drugs Affecting Women's Health and the Female Reproductive System

1. synthetic hormone chemically identical to natural luteinizing hormone–releasing hormone; the synthesis and release of LH and FSH
2. a fixed ratio of estrogen and progestin taken for 21 days of normal menstrual cycle; least
3. follicular; luteal
4. normal estrogen and progesterone levels during the menstrual cycle
5. ovulation; abnormal bleeding or infertility
6. C, A, A, A, A, A, C, A, A, A, A, A and C
7. Take basal temperature daily and record from day 1 of menstrual period and every morning upon awakening. Coitus should occur every other day for 3 to 4 days before ovulation and 2 to 3 days after ovulation. Take the medication at the same time every day. If the medication is to start on day 5, count the first day of the menstrual period as day 1.

If a dose is missed, advise client to take it as soon as possible. If dose is not remembered until time for the next dose, both should be taken together. If more than one dose is missed, consult physician. Report abdominal pain or visual disturbance immediately. Be cautious with tasks that require alertness.

Chapter 53: Drugs for Labor and Delivery

1. contraction of the smooth muscle of the uterus; contractions and spontaneous labor
2. labor that occurs before the thirty-seventh week of pregnancy; 10 to 15
3. several prior births
4. Most frequent: nausea or vomiting, mostly after IV administration. Less frequent: diarrhea, dizziness, tinnitus, increased sweating, confusion. Dose-related effect: abdominal cramping.
5. Used investigationally for the inhibition of premature labor
6. Checking the pulse before boluses are delivered, keeping prefilled syringes cool and protected from light when stored, and protecting the pump from moisture and from being dropped. Proper disposal of used syringes and infusion sets is also covered.
7. Fluid volume excess (pulmonary edema); altered comfort related to headache, or nausea and vomiting; impaired skin integrity related to rash; anxiety (restlessness, nervousness, emotional lability); the collaborative problems of increased cardiac output (tachycardia), which could result in angina, myocardial infarction, and cardiac dysrhythmias and hepatitis.

1. Word search key:

```
U  T  K  P  N  I  I  B  G  E  G  C  C  O  D  I  B  I  L
T  B  A  V  R  R  D  P  F  N  E  I  U  Y  V  L  S  W  Y
P  S  S  R  G  G  Z  H  C  C  I  T  F  Q  F  B  S  W  O
T  Q  J  Z  C  R  H  M  N  A  S  S  E  S  S  M  E  N  T
H  A  C  F  N  O  E  K  U  P  E  A  R  N  S  L  N  A  M
T  Q  H  S  L  Y  V  C  U  I  D  L  W  U  H  Q  I  A  D
V  R  A  B  P  L  Z  B  P  N  I  P  J  Q  N  F  Z  I  E
J  C  F  D  R  M  E  A  N  D  R  O  G  E  N  S  Z  T  P
L  U  C  J  O  R  L  N  A  I  E  E  E  K  H  M  I  S  R
E  P  D  H  T  M  L  E  Y  C  T  N  C  Z  R  E  D  A  E
M  R  O  Y  E  X  M  M  S  A  S  I  I  N  E  R  J  M  S
I  O  N  N  I  Q  X  I  P  T  A  T  D  P  A  E  Q  O  S
D  S  T  I  N  D  Q  A  C  I  N  N  N  U  C  C  X  C  I
W  T  Y  H  V  J  S  U  X  O  I  A  U  R  T  T  S  E  O
O  A  X  S  D  B  T  T  Z  N  F  O  A  R  I  I  X  N  N
Y  T  B  L  D  D  O  X  V  S  C  U  J  N  O  O  V  Y  K
T  E  S  T  O  S  T  E  R  O  N  E  I  X  N  N  A  G  O
F  U  J  A  I  A  M  P  Y  R  S  D  B  G  S  S  Q  Y  K
O  V  O  U  Z  O  O  H  Y  P  O  G  O  N  A  D  I  S  M
```

2. Treatment of androgen deficiency; treatment of delayed male puberty when not induced by a pathologic condition; treatment of breast carcinoma; anemia

3. With oral anticoagulants, anticoagulant effects may be enhanced or increased; with other hepatotoxic medications, the risk of inducing hepatotoxicity is increased.

4. Disturbance in self-concept; fluid volume excess; altered comfort related to nausea, vomiting, and abdominal pain; altered sleep pattern; potential complications of erythrocytosis, hepatic impairment, hypercalcemia, and polycythemia

5. benign prostatic hyperplasia; the glandular and connective tissue in the portions of the prostate that surround the urethra

6. Decreased libido, impotence, decreased amount of ejaculate

Chapter 55: Drugs Affecting Sexual Behavior

1. sexual drive
2. transudation
3. achieve; maintain
4. anxiety; irritability; depression; premenstrual syndrome
5. libido; potency
6. *Antidepressants, antihypertensives:* impotence
   Diuretics, H_2 receptors: impotence, gynecomastia
   Antianxiety drugs, alcohol, barbiturates: impotence, decreased sexual activity
7. Gaining understanding and acceptance of feelings about one's own sexuality; being open to clients' discussions; allowing clients to hold any belief or sexual practice that is not overtly harmful; recognizing that it is probably impossible to be truly comfortable with all clients or topics; keeping current

with constantly changing data about drugs with potential for causing sexual dysfunction; being able to identify and interpret client cues about problems dealing with sexuality; discussing clients' medication with them; consulting with prescriber when adverse reactions appear and suggesting alternate forms, if feasible; listening with sensitivity to expressed feelings that may attend body image changes.

Chapter 56: Principles of Antineoplastic Chemotherapy

1. generic; over 300 defined disease states; cardiovascular disease
2. metastasis
3. cytologic; carcinoma of cervix and endometrium in subclinical stages
4. adverse; the maximum permissible dose has been delivered; the drug needs to be discontinued
5. Growth pattern of tumor in which tumor enlarges, nearly outgrows its blood and nutrient supply, and the growth rate pattern decreases or plateaus.
6. *G1 phase:* phase of cell reproduction in which RNA and protein synthesis may occur
   S phase: replication phase of cell reproduction in which DNA doubles
   G2 phase: postsynthesis or premitotic phase of cell reproduction in which DNA synthesis ceases while RNA and protein synthesis continues
   M phase: mitotic phase of cell reproduction in which cells divide into two completely new cells that may leave the cell cycle
7. *GI tract:* nausea, vomiting, anorexia, diarrhea
   Bone marrow: bone marrow suppression
   Hair follicles: alopecia (hair loss)
   Mouth: stomatitis (inflammation of the mouth)
8. *Constipation:* addition to diet of high-fiber foods and prune juice, 1-2 tbsp of bran, 8-10 glasses of fluid daily, and/or hot lemon water in the morning.
   Alopecia: assure client that hair will begin to grow back in 6 to 8 weeks, although it may be a different texture or color.
   Stomatitis: good oral hygiene; small, frequent servings of cold or room-temperature, bland, nonirritating foods. Choice of mouthwash depends on status of client's lesions.
9. They should be handled with gloves, emptied directly into toilet, washed with detergent and water without splashing with the rinse water discarded directly into toilet, and the toilet flushed three times.

Chapter 57: Antineoplastic Chemotherapy Agents

1. interfering with cell reproduction or replication at some point in cell cycle
2. a necessary building block for formation of DNA; normal production of DNA
3. an alkyl chemical structure; a hydrogen atom
4. DNA functioning; blocking the transcription of new DNA or RNA
5. plant alkaloids; cell division in metaphase
6. time that sensitive (normal) cells are exposed to toxic effects of methotrexate
7.

Antineoplastic drug	Action
fluorouracil	Interferes with synthesis of DNA and RNA
mechlorethamine	Prevents cell division and protein synthesis
doxorubicin	Binds DNA and inhibits RNA synthesis
vinblastine, vincristine	Inhibits mitosis during M-phase
interferon	Inhibits virus replication, decreases cell proliferation, and enhances phagocyte activity
paclitaxel	Produces stable microtubule bundles and interferes with the late G-2 mitotic phase in cell cycle

8. c, a, b, d
9. Apply topical cooling via the following steps:
   (1) Cooling of site to client tolerance for 24 hours.
   (2) Elevate and rest extremity for 24 to 48 hours, then resume normal activity as tolerated.
   (3) If pain, erythema, and/or swelling persist beyond 48 hours, discuss with the physician the need for consultation with surgeon.

Chapter 58: Overview of Infections, Inflammation, and Fever

1. See Fig. 58-1, which provides an overview of heat loss and heat gain mechanisms.
2. c, d, a, b, d, d, c, a
3. Teach that these drugs should never be taken without medical supervision and should be taken in strict accordance with physicians' prescriptions. Allergic clients should be taught to protect themselves from future exposure. Special administration

considerations, expected effects, side effects, and adverse reactions can be described on drug sheets for clients to refer to at home, with a telephone number to call when questions arise. Caution client that occasionally these drugs will interfere with results of home lab testing kits.

Chapter 59: Antibiotics

1. kill; suppress; microorganisms; penicillins; cephalosporins; macrolide antibiotics; quinolones
2. penicillins
3. Refer to Fig. 3-7, p. 45, in the textbook.
4. The peak and trough determine the pharmacokinetics of an antibiotic and help determine dosage and intervals of administration.
5.

Antibiotic	Side effects to monitor
chloramphenicol	Diarrhea, nausea, vomiting
erythromycin	Diarrhea, nausea, vomiting; soreness of tongue and mouth; abdominal distress
clindamycin	Most frequent: mild diarrhea, skin rash Less frequent: pruritus of skin, rectum, genital area
ciprofloxacin	Nausea, diarrhea, vomiting, headache, skin rash, stomach upset, restlessness
lincomycin	Most frequent: mild diarrhea, skin rash Less frequent: pruritus of skin, rectum, genital area
vancomycin	Oral dosage form: nausea, vomiting, taste alterations Parenteral dosage form: none

6. T, F, F
7. Refer to the box on p. 986 of your textbook for a complete listing.

Chapter 60: Antifungal and Antiviral Drugs

1. *Candida albicans;* pruritus; white exudate; peeling; easy bleeding of tissue
2. plantlike; parasitic
3. infections; fungi
4. chemoprophylaxis
5. Advise client to complete essential dental work before starting therapy with amphotericin B or to delay it until completing course of drug to avoid gingival bleeding and delayed healing. Teach appropriate oral hygiene, including gentle use of soft toothbrushes and floss and avoidance of toothpicks. Advise client to alert staff at first indication of pain at IV site.
6. In viral diseases, by the time signs and symptoms appear, multiplication of the virus is ending. To be clinically effective, antiviral drugs must be administered chemoprophylactically.
7. *Alcohol:* increased risk for CNS side effects such as dizziness, fainting, etc.
   Anticholinergics: increase in anticholinergic side effects such as hallucinations, dry mouth, etc.
   CNS-stimulating agents: increased CNS stimulation; cardiac dysrhythmias and convulsions may occur.
8. Nausea, myalgia, insomnia, severe headache, bone marrow suppression
9. Administer on empty stomach. Tablets should not be swallowed whole but thoroughly chewed, crushed, or dissolved in water. Dissolve in at least 30 ml of water, stir, and have client swallow it immediately.

Chapter 61: Other Antimicrobial Drugs and Antiparasitic Drugs

1. Word search key:

```
D  J  G  R  U  H  D  S  I  S  O  L  U  C  R  E  B  U  T  Y
L  W  N  X  D  D  G  I  P  A  T  H  O  G  E  N  E  S  I  S
I  M  I  H  R  Y  P  F  Z  R  M  P  I  T  G  I  R  S  G  X
Y  K  S  W  V  D  Y  X  M  A  L  A  R  I  A  P  V  I  T  Z
O  Y  R  V  J  V  T  L  W  T  I  R  C  A  F  M  E  S  O  X
L  T  U  E  T  I  S  A  R  A  P  N  E  P  U  A  D  A  X  L
A  E  N  I  U  Q  O  R  O  L  H  C  O  Y  R  F  I  I  O  F
M  F  O  E  R  Y  T  H  R  O  C  Y  T  I  C  I  M  N  P  O
E  A  T  R  C  O  M  M  U  N  I  T  Y  O  N  R  A  O  L  W
B  S  F  N  P  H  Y  D  D  G  E  C  E  R  S  S  N  M  A  O
I  M  L  B  V  N  I  H  A  B  B  F  C  H  P  E  I  O  S  U
A  M  I  N  O  S  A  L  I  C  Y  L  A  T  E  Y  Z  H  M  X
S  I  L  Y  E  N  D  P  D  U  H  Q  E  S  Q  J  A  C  O  T
I  F  Y  A  S  K  U  L  Z  R  C  T  L  G  D  P  R  I  S  B
S  U  S  E  E  Z  C  Q  P  R  E  G  N  A  N  C  Y  R  I  T
G  E  N  E  D  U  C  A  T  I  O  N  K  A  U  R  P  T  S  K
J  A  S  U  O  T  A  M  O  L  U  N  A  R  G  S  M  F  A  K
H  E  L  M  I  N  T  H  S  M  R  O  W  N  I  P  L  N  D  V
D  L  D  W  L  T  S  K  S  G  V  Q  S  A  T  E  D  B  B  Q
Q  O  G  F  V  L  J  Y  K  J  F  O  B  L  J  G  Z  K  G  B
```

2. Refer to opening section of the chapter for a complete description.
3. Transmitted by airborne droplets, not by objects. Sharing enclosed environment with infected person creates high risk of developing this infection.
4. Monitor client's response to therapy. Ensure client adherence. Monitor for adverse drug reactions.
5. Encourage compliance with full course of drug. Regular visits and periodic eye examinations are necessary. Report vision changes promptly. Do not use alcohol and oral antacids with isoniazid. Drug may produce false-positive test results with copper sulfate tests. Clients should use other urine glucose tests.
6. Major side effects include nausea, vomiting, stomach cramps, diarrhea, headaches, dizziness, ataxia, trembling, muscle weakness, paresthesia, convulsions, memory defect, blurred vision, nystagmus and other visual disturbances, and hypersensitivity (rash, hives, fever, cough, bronchospasm, lacrimation).

Chapter 62: Overview of the Immunologic System

1. b, c, d — a — b, c, d — b — a — b — c, d — a — c, d — b
2. circulate in the blood in an inactive form; activated in precise order
3. *IgG:* the most abundant and major immunoglobulin; can enter all areas of tissues
   IgM: first immunoglobulin during an immune response; activates the complement system
   IgA: located in the external body secretions; provides defense on exposed surfaces
   IgD: is in plasma and on lymphocyte surfaces; function is unknown

IgE: binds to histamine-containing mast cells and basophils; mediates release of histamine

4. Consult Table 62-1, p. 1078 in the textbook, for the correct answers.

Chapter 63: Serums, Vaccines, and Other Immunizing Agents

1. the concentration of antibodies in the serum; disease exposure and immunity
2. diphtheria-pertussis-tetanus vaccine
3. trivalent oral poliovirus vaccine
4. measles-mumps-rubella vaccine
5. passive immunization
6. Answers should include two of the following issues: Live vaccine–related diseases have surfaced as problems.
   Increasingly, a college-age person or parent is the subject of a relatively virulent form of some childhood disease for which he or she was immunized much earlier or whose antibody titers are waning.
   Other secondary effects are surfacing: some booster injections seem to increase sensitivity to antigen, with severe reactions.
   Poultry allergy is less of a potential threat than originally supposed.
   Evidence is building that desired antibody formation from vaccines is subject to interference from concurrent passive transfer by various routes.
7. Relative safety and merits of immunization versus risk of disease itself should be discussed. Client and/or family should be told that repeat immunization is usually not contraindicated when records are unclear. Unimmunized parents should be identified and probably immunized before their children, especially when TOPV is administered.
   Noncompletion of an immunization series may occasionally be prevented if vaccinees or parents know that interruption makes no difference to eventual antibody levels. Copy of schedule enhances compliance. Teach parents or vaccinees to keep careful written records and bring them to each appointment.
8. P, P, A, A, P, A, P, A, P, A, P, A

Chapter 64: Immunosuppressants and Immunomodulators

1. decrease; prevent; azathioprine; cyclosporine; muromonab-CD3
2. severe combined immune deficiency syndrome
3. diminished

4. human immunodeficiency virus; AIDS
5. the body's immune defenses; biologic response to unwanted stimulus
6. It is believed that HIV is a retrovirus that has RNA in its core. After it binds to CD4+ T-lymphocyte receptor cells, it releases its RNA into the cytoplasm. Reverse transcriptase assists in transcribing the HIV RNA into viral DNA strands in host body. Thereafter, activation of this DNA results in production of viral substances that infect other CD4+ T-lymphocyte cells. The CD4+ helper cells are destroyed by the virus, which leads to AIDS.
7. Increased hair growth and trembling. With long-term therapy: dose-dependent nephrotoxicity, severe hypertension, lymphomas and other lymphoproliferative-type disorders, gingival hyperplasia.
8. Refer to *Nursing Management: The Immunosuppressed Client* for complete list of possible answers.
9. Consult Box 64-1, p. 1105 in the textbook, for a complete list.

Chapter 65: Overview of the Integumentary System

1. Refer to Fig. 65-1, p. 1116, in the textbook.
2. Sebaceous, eccrine, apocrine
3. 4.5 to 5.5 (weakly acidic)
4. Protective function; organ of sensation; body temperature regulator; excretion of fluid and electrolytes; storage of fat; synthesizing vitamin D; site for drug absorption; contributes to body image and feeling of well-being

Chapter 66: Dermatologic Drugs

1. b, e, c, b, a, d, f, c, a, c, b, f, e, e, d, e, d
2. Baths, soaps, solutions and lotions, cleansers, emollients, skin protectants, wet dressings and soaks, rubs, liniments
3. Impaired skin integrity; altered comfort related to pain, burning, or itching of affected areas; risk for infection related to open skin areas; self-care deficits related to location of affected areas; knowledge deficit related to new or altered dermatologic therapy; disturbance in self-concept related to perceived and actual disfigurement of affected areas

Chapter 67: Debriding Agents

1. Cryptoquote: Many causes contribute to decubitus ulcers.

2. Delayed healing; increased risk of bacterial infection; allergic or sensitivity reactions.

With collagenase: transient erythema. With fibrinolysin and desoxyribonuclease: allergic reactions in persons sensitive to bovine sources, mercury compounds, or chloramphenicol. With sutilains: mild transient pain, local paresthesia, bleeding, transient dermatitis

3. *Stage I or II:* silicone spray, transparent or hydrocolloidal dressing

Stage III: wet to dry dressings, enzymatic debridement, hydrocolloidal dressing

Stage IV: wet to dry dressings, enzymatic debridement, surgical debridement

4. Refer to list on pp. 1140-1143 for complete coverage of interventions.

Chapter 68: Vitamins and Minerals

1. nutrition challenge; rapid growth; pregnancy; lactation; convalescence
2. avitaminosis
3. vitamin C
4. A, D, E, K

5.

Vitamin	Other names or chemical names
A	retinol, the carotenes
B_1	thiamine
B_2	riboflavin
B_3	niacin
B_6	pyridoxine
B_9	folic acid
B_{12}	cyanocobalamin
C	ascorbic acid, sodium ascorbate
D	calcifediol, calcitriol, dihydrotachysterol, ergocalciferol
E	alpha-tocopherol

6. Recommended daily allowance
7. Alert client that iron preparations cause black stools, which are medically insignificant. However, client should report other symptoms of internal blood loss. Instruct client to maintain diet rich in sources of iron such as liver, green leafy vegetables, potatoes, dried peas and beans, dried fruit, and enriched flour, bread, and cereals.

Chapter 69: Fluids and Electrolytes

1. c — e, f — d — a — b — g — e — b, f — a — h
2. Potassium (K+), magnesium (Mg++)
3. Sodium (Na+), chloride (Cl-), bicarbonate (HCO_3-)
4.

Category	Solution	Use
Hydrating solution	Dextrose 2.5%, 5%, or higher in water; dextrose in 0.2% or 0.5% normal saline	To hydrate or prevent dehydration; to assess kidney status before electrolyte therapy; to help increase diuresis in dehydrated individuals
Isotonic solution	Isotonic chloride; Ringer's injection; lactated Ringer's injection	To replace extracellular fluid losses in which chloride loss ≥ sodium loss; isotonic or normal saline: before and after blood transfusion; isotonic sodium chloride: to treat metabolic alkalosis
Maintenance solution	Plasma-Lyte; Normosol	To replace daily electrolyte and extracellular needs and water; to replace electrolytes and water loss from severe vomiting or diarrhea

5. c, b, a, c, c, b, c, a
6. Ensure that only health care providers, fully prepared in EID technology, be authorized to set up, adjust, or remove IV administration sets. Check that infusion is not running when pump is removed. Check or recalculate infusion rate. Apply visible labels to EIDs that do not prevent free flow to alert staff. Limit use of one type of EID to each unit. Use only protected EIDs in CCUs or with critical care drugs.

Chapter 70: Enteral and Parenteral Nutrition

1. oral; tube; nasogastric; nasoduodenal; esophagostomic; gastrostomy; jejunostomy
2. total parenteral nutrition (TPN); intravenous; complete nutrition
3. promote production of proteins; reduce protein breakdown; help promote wound healing
4. synthesized by the body
5. Refer to Table 70-2 for possible answers.
6. Refer to *Nursing Management: Parenteral Nutrition Therapy* section for full coverage of possible answers.
7. Preparation of client and family member should begin 5 to 7 days before discharge. Teach signs of incorrect tube placement and insertion and removal if needed. Written and verbal instructions on possible complications are also necessary. Understanding of procedure, rationale, and expectations of tube feedings can aid in active client participation and greater satisfaction.
8. Catheter seeding from blood-borne or distant infection; contamination of catheter entrance site during insertion or long-term catheter placement; solution contamination

Chapter 71: Antiseptics, Disinfectants, and Sterilants

1. a hospital; urinary tract; postoperative wound
2. pathogenic organisms; all microorganisms; reduce number and spread of organisms
3. all forms of life; an instrument or utensil; a liquid; a substance; living tissue
4. nonliving objects; living tissue; less potent; more dilute
5. Handwashing
6. They may change the structure of the protein of the microbial cell; lower the surface tension of the aqueous medium of the parasitic cell; interfere with some metabolic processes of the microbial cell in such ways as to interfere with the cell's ability to survive and multiply.
7. Chiefly used to treat minor wounds, abrasions, and infected wounds and for indwelling urethral catheter care, skin preparation before invasive procedures, Hickman catheter and parenteral nutrition dressing changes, and IV needle insertions. They are also used for disinfecting indwelling catheters for peritoneal dialysis and for sanitizing water and air. An aqueous solution of 5% iodine and 10% potassium iodide can also be given orally to treat goiter.
8. Do not bandage or tape areas treated with tincture of iodine; if treated with povidone-iodine, cover dressing may be applied. If irritation develops, wash the skin. Artificially elevated blood glucose determinations have been noted when povidone-iodine swabs were used for skin preparation. Soap and water cleansing of fingertips before skin puncture for blood glucose monitoring by some reagent strips is recommended. Iodophors will stain only starched linen or clothing. Tinctures and solutions of iodine may stain more freely.
9. Store in tightly capped, amber containers; solutions in containers should be discarded frequently and fresh solutions used. Bubbling action makes hydrogen peroxide useful for removing mucous secretions from equipment. Do not leave paper cups of hydrogen peroxide in client's reach, since it may be mistaken for water. Keep these compounds secured and out of reach of children.

Chapter 72: Diagnostic Agents

1. Word search key:

```
S N O I T A C I D N I  G L R B E G G N G H
D E S S E R P P U S O N U M M I C N N I U
L R U M B F N E G T N E O R T F Q I D U U
S G P S X Y V T D C M Y I C H A X N Q Y L
M X O C F Y Z A A O T H Z W G F J O B D T
I M K R Q Z B W N N R P Z N K R R I E D R
R L N E C R V X T T E A Y N J G V T M I A
P A Y E B N Q V I R A R R B A B E C B A S
R T D N X X T D H A T G G N U C P N F G O
A O S I W U M W I S M O S Y T E I U L N N
D M R N O Z M D S T E I R I I A N F U O G
I O T G U A M R T C N G O L K D E H S S G
O G C W T R C V A N T N M D A F P I H T R
N R N B V Y S T M D V A U J K F H T I I A
U A S U S A G I I T I L T C S S R W N C P
C P I B X Q G W N V L O N G H X I U G S H
L H N X S D R R E G E H P Y J X N Q E A Y
I Y G F S R F K S O F C C A Z A E R P J H
D A Q E X Z F F W G K L E F Q M J U M B G
E U R A D I O P H A R M A C E U T I C A L
S X V V I S U A L I Z A T I O N E B H E H
```

2. Refer to Table 72-5 for complete listing.
3. Refer to Table 72-3 for complete listing.
4. Refer to *Intervention* under *Nursing Management: Radiopaque Agents* for answer.

Chapter 73: Poisons and Antidotes

1. poisons; their action and effects; methods of detection; diagnosis and treatment of poisoning
2. relatively small; death; serious bodily harm
3. clusters of signs associated with common drug poisonings or overdoses
4. emetic; bittersweet
5. narcotic emetic; reflex action of the vomiting center in the brainstem
6. washing out of the stomach
7. emesis; lavage; an absorbent
8. organophosphate intoxication; Salivation; Lacrimation; Urination; Defecation; Gastrointestinal distress; Emesis
9. Attain quick assessment and history to determine extent of impairments or particular susceptibilities. Observe vital signs and level of consciousness.
   Implementation may include turning, deep breathing, coughing, suctioning, and auscultation to demonstrate need for chest x-ray, suctioning, tracheostomy, endotracheal intubation, blood gas determinations, supplemental oxygen, and a respirator/ventilator.
   Position victim to prevent aspiration; attend mouth care promptly after emesis. Moderate amounts of plain water by mouth may dilute or effectively inactivate many ingested poisons.
10. d, a, e, b, f, c